Promoting Mobility for
People with Dementia

A problem-solving approach

Rosemary Oddy

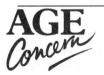

BOOKS

© 1998 Rosemary Oddy
Published by Age Concern England
1268 London Road
London SW16 4ER

First published 1998
Editor Gillian Clarke
Design and typesetting GreenGate Publishing Services
Production Vinnette Marshall
Printed in Great Britain by Bell & Bain Ltd, Glasgow

A catalogue record for this book is available from the British Library

ISBN 0–86242–242–6

Bulk orders
Age Concern England is pleased to offer customised editions of all its titles to UK companies, institutions or other organisations wishing to make a bulk purchase. For further information, please contact the Publishing Department at the address on this page. Tel: 0181-679 8000. Fax: 0181-679 6069. E-mail: addisom@ace.org.uk

Contents

About the author

Rosemary is the former head of Leicestershire's mental health physiotherapy service, and was one of the first Chartered physiotherapists to be employed in a psychiatric hospital in the UK.

She spent 27 years working at the Carlton Hayes Hospital in Leicestershire, adapting her physiotherapy skills to suit the needs of the many different patients. She particularly enjoyed treating older people and developed a very special interest in those with dementia. Since retiring from the National Health Service in 1994, Rosemary has been able to concentrate on sharing her experience and ideas with colleagues and carers at home and overseas.

Acknowledgements

I acknowledge with thanks the contribution of the physiotherapists who worked with me in the early 'pioneering' days; Elizabeth Douglas and Heather Freegard of the Sir James McCusker Training Foundation in Perth, Western Australia, for persuading me to write the book; colleagues, Barbara Sutcliffe and Brian Fletcher for reviewing the manuscript; and my husband, David, for his patient support and encouragement.

Introduction: why a book about mobility?

You can read about dementia in many books and gain valuable advice about caring and managing the problems of people in your care. There is, however, very little written about the important subject of promoting or maintaining mobility. When the subject is mentioned, many authors give the impression that they expect people with dementia to become bed-bound. Some authors talk briefly about the importance of exercise, giving physical help and the possible use of walking aids, but there is very little detail to guide you.

This book is devoted entirely to the subject of promoting and maintaining mobility, and is full of problem-solving ideas. If you are determined to succeed and are willing to meet the challenge, you can achieve some surprisingly satisfying results.

Who can make use of the book?

Qualified nurses and care workers and their assistants, student therapists and nurses, qualified therapists new to this field of work and carers (see Glossary) should find in it much that provokes thought and action. Other professional workers such as psychologists, social workers and medical staff, who need a patient to move for them, will also benefit from using some of the suggested strategies. And finally, it should be of interest to managers of residential or nursing establishments who provide services for people with dementia, and to those who design or plan the layout of the buildings used by them.

Using the book

There is a great deal of information and a wealth of ideas in this book for you to put into practice. Each chapter contains details of a range of strategies that you can use for the problems being discussed. The strategies are made up of different approaches or methods, giving you ways of overcoming or easing some of the problems that you encounter during your daily work. They cannot guarantee a particular result, but they do provide you with many pieces for the mobility 'jigsaw'. Study the pieces carefully so that you know how they fit together.

Note If you have not received training in giving physical help, you will need guidance from a physiotherapist or occupational therapist before you use some of the strategies (see 'Gaining access to help and advice' on p 88).

At the end of most chapters there are some useful training exercises. They are designed to help you to understand better the difficulties experienced by people with dementia and to give you the opportunity to try out some of the strategies that you can use.

Planning your reading

It will take you time to read and re-read the chapters and carry out the suggested exercises. It might be a good idea to scan the whole book quickly to gain a general impression and then to study each chapter in detail afterwards. You could also use the points raised in each chapter as topics for discussion with your colleagues and practise the relevant strategies afterwards.

Using the lists of strategies

Appendix 2 gives lists of strategies that have been used successfully to help to promote or maintain a particular activity. They are there for you to copy and use, and to add to.

Introducing you to the people named in the book

People with dementia receive support and care in a variety of different settings: some are able to remain in their own homes, while others are cared for in residential or nursing homes. You will meet four of them – fictional people who represent my experiences from these different settings. Mr Rajeev Patel, Miss Ruth Kenny, Mr Harry Cash and Mrs Anna Polanszky have some of the mobility problems that may affect people with dementia.

Mr Rajeev Patel, aged 91 years, lives in a small modernised terraced house with his wife. He is a small, frail, wiry man and has multi-infarct dementia (see Chapter 1) – he has had coronary heart disease (see Glossary) for many years. He is cared for at home by his 72-year-old wife who has access to advice from a community psychiatric nurse. Mr Patel is aware of his condition and sometimes becomes very agitated and angry. Mrs Patel manages her husband very well and is anxious to keep him mobile as long as possible. She is an intelligent, good-natured woman who enjoys good health.

Mr Patel was for many years sub-postmaster of the post office near their home, and his wife helped him in the adjacent shop. They are both respected members of their local community.

Miss Ruth Kenny is 66 years old and a retired secondary school teacher. She was given early retirement on grounds of ill-health at the age of 57. She suffered with high blood-pressure. During her working life she was very particular about her personal appearance and dressed smartly.

Miss Kenny was admitted to a local authority nursing home recently after several incidents in her maisonette. Action had to be taken when she set her kitchen on fire – she placed a newspaper over a lighted burner on the gas stove. She had become increasingly forgetful and unkempt. She has been diagnosed as having dementia. She has no relatives, but an ex-teaching colleague visits her regularly.

Mr Harry Cash, a widower, is 85 years old. He worked as a full-time fireman until his retirement. His wife died many years ago and he did not remarry. Their only son emigrated to Australia, where he set up home and married an English girl out there. The young couple never managed to persuade Mr Cash to join them, but they have always kept in close touch and his son has returned a couple of times to visit him.

Mr Cash, a keen gardener, remained active and in relatively good health until two years ago. He then started to suffer from small strokes and became increasingly depressed and inactive. After some investigations, he was diagnosed as having multi-infarct dementia. Until recently, he was supported at home by good neighbours and by a home carer scheme paid for by his son. Three months ago, it was decided that he needed constant care, so his son arranged for him to be admitted to a private nursing home. Mr Cash agreed to this and settled down very well. His mobility is deteriorating and he moves only when he is asked to.

Mrs Anna Polanszky is 72 years of age and is suffering from dementia of Alzheimer's type (see Chapter 1). She came to England from Poland as a young married woman at the beginning of the second world war. After serving in the war, her husband set up a small printing business which became very successful. Mrs Polanszky did not have to go out to work; she stayed at home and devoted herself to her family and her husband. She never learnt to speak English fluently.

Mrs Polanszky was admitted to a residential home six months ago, shortly after her husband died. She was deeply shocked and distressed by his death – she neglected herself and refused any help. Mrs Polanszky is a heavily built woman with painful arthritic knees and for some time has moved with difficulty. She is inclined to be bad-tempered.

Other people In addition to these four named people, who are used to illustrate particular points in the text, you will meet others. In order to avoid confusion when describing them and the people caring for them, and to simplify explanations when general comments are made, *unnamed people with dementia will be referred to as males, and care staff as females.*

1 Dementia and Mobility Problems

This chapter begins with a brief description of the most common types of dementia. It then looks at ways in which people's abilities and behaviour are affected and how these in their turn can affect mobility. Consideration is also given to the physical conditions that can trouble any older person, and which can interfere with mobility.

Types of dementia

Dementia is not part of the normal ageing process. The term is used to describe the set of symptoms caused by a group of diseases. You are most likely to meet people who are thought to have *dementia of the Alzheimer's type* or *vascular dementia*, of which *multi-infarct dementia* is the commonest type. Statistics show that 6 per cent of people over the age of 65, and 20 per cent of those over the age of 80, have some form of dementia (Department of Health 1995).

Dementia causes a progressive decline in intellectual ability and affects memory and the ability to carry out the physical activities of daily living (World Health Organization 1990). This decline is sometimes accompanied by changes in personality and a deterioration in social behaviour. The changes in the brain are permanent and cannot be reversed.

Dementia of Alzheimer's type

This most common type of dementia usually starts very gradually. It accounts for about 50 per cent of all dementias that occur. Another 10 per cent have a mixed type of dementia, involving dementia of Alzheimer's type and multi-infarct dementia. Memory is often affected first but, because we all tend to be forgetful at times, it is almost impossible to pinpoint the onset. You should not jump to the conclusion that someone has dementia just because their memory is not as good as it was. The diagnosis is made by a doctor, who carefully rules out all the other possible explanations before doing so. Questionnaire-type tests are available to help doctors identify people who are suffering from depression rather than dementia.

It is now known that some families are more prone to dementia than others. This applies to both early *and* late onset forms of the disease. Dementia of Alzheimer's type that starts before the age of 65 is considered to be an early onset dementia; it is possible for people as young as 45 years to develop it.

Vascular dementia

Diseases of the body's blood vessels are responsible for the onset of vascular dementia. One such condition, called arteriosclerosis, involves a 'hardening' of the arteries. This means that the supply of blood to the brain may not be as good as it should be, and in some cases it can be cut off. People who suffer from arteriosclerosis may also suffer from high blood pressure and heart disease.

Vascular dementias are thought to account for about 20 per cent of all types of dementia. The most common vascular dementia is the type called *multi-infarct dementia*. In this, the person's condition gradually becomes worse as a result of many small strokes. So, instead of the steady worsening seen in dementia of Alzheimer's type, it usually occurs in a series of steps. The other feature of multi-infarct dementia that you need to be aware of is the likelihood of fluctuations or variations in people's performance. Their ability to communicate and carry out everyday activities may vary from day to day, or even from hour to hour. This is not due to any deliberate action on their part, but is caused by variations in the blood flow to the brain.

Other dementias

The remaining 20 per cent of dementias are caused by a variety of other conditions. These include Parkinson's disease, Lewy body disease (see Glossary), AIDS and alcoholism. You are very likely to meet people who suffer from Parkinsonism (see Glossary) – they feel rather stiff when you help them, and they find it particularly difficult to start moving.

How do people react to having dementia?

As the dementia progresses, people are gradually robbed of a great deal of their intellectual, physical and social abilities. Some react with flashes of aggression, while others become withdrawn and sad. You will also find that some people are more aware than others of these losses. Those with vascular dementia are more likely to realise what is happening to them than are those who have dementia of Alzheimer's type. It is not hard to imagine our own initial anger or sadness if we had to face such a diagnosis: 'Why me?', 'What have I done to deserve this?'

Some of these people become clinically *depressed*. They need to be treated for depression and to be encouraged to maintain a reasonable level of activity – people who are depressed do not want to move. Older people with depression can 'go off their feet' very quickly, especially if they already have painful arthritic hips and knees or other conditions that make movement difficult.

What is mobility?

The term *mobility* can mean different things to different people. In this book it is used to describe the daily activities that enable us to move about in our surroundings:

- rising to standing;
- walking;
- sitting down;
- moving from one seat to another;
- moving on and off the bed;
- climbing and going down stairs.

How dementia affects mobility

We now need to take a look at the losses, or *impairments*, caused by dementia. These impairments are examined under a series of different headings so that you can see how they affect mobility.

Memory

People with dementia may set out to sit on a chair a short distance away but fail to reach it – they forget what they are doing or where they are going. Worse still, they may try to stand up or get out of bed – forgetting that they cannot do either without help – and fall. Their memory may be so poor that they forget what they have been asked to do after only a very few seconds. You may see them preparing to carry out the movement, then forgetting it, and they settle down again.

The experts tell us that there are different types of memory. People who are unable to remember what you are asking them to do may well be able to tell you some interesting tales from their youth. This is because their short-term memory is impaired by dementia, but their long-term memory is less likely to be affected.

Thinking

We are able to follow instructions that guide us through movements in a variety of different directions. If we are asked, for example, to move *up* or to move *sideways*, we instantly think about what is required and do it. People with dementia find this type of thinking difficult or impossible. They may, therefore, not understand a similar request, although they are able to carry it out. Chapter 3 suggests different ways of helping them to understand the direction of the movements you ask them to do.

You also need to be aware that people with dementia may not be able to carry out a movement if they have to think about it. This is because, when we carry out familiar or well practised movements, we do so more or less automatically. It is only when we are learning something new or when we are paying particular attention to detail that we have to think about the movement. The strategies that you can use to encourage people to move at an automatic level are described in Chapter 7.

Orientation

People with dementia often lose their ability to keep track of time and of their whereabouts. Some are inclined to live in the past. So when you ask them to accompany you, they may politely refuse, and give you a very convincing reason why they cannot go with you. Unless you know something of their past and present pattern of life, you may find it difficult to decide whether the reason given is a valid one. It is important not to allow their confusion between the past and the present to deprive them of some essential activity.

Changes of position can cause fear and distress – people with dementia become *disorientated* rather easily, so you should always give them plenty of time to adjust to a change of position.

Communication

Some people with dementia may have difficulty in finding the right words to speak. This means that it is difficult for them to tell you that they want your help to move, or that they are in pain and therefore unwilling to move. Others may be very slow, or have great difficulty in understanding what you are asking them to do. So give them plenty of time to try to understand, and repeat what you said to them. Chapters 2 and 3 suggest ways in which you can talk to people you are caring for.

Learning

It is not easy for people with dementia to learn new skills. They are, however, able to carry out some new activities. For example, they can learn to use a walking aid, especially if it can be wheeled. Nevertheless, you will usually need to prompt them to use it and to position it correctly. So the walking aid may make it possible for them to walk without your physical support, but it does not necessarily mean that they can do so without your being there. To be independent they need to be able to motivate themselves to move and to find their own way about – many of them cannot do this.

Judgement

Throughout the course of our lives we learn from our experiences. This gives us the ability to foresee the likely consequences of particular actions and to avoid making the same mistakes too many times. People with dementia may lose much of this ability, so they make misjudgements that can affect their own safety and that of others. For example, one frail person may attempt to help another to walk, and they both fall.

And some people misjudge their distance from the chair they are approaching – they either just manage to land on the seat or finish up on the floor (see Chapter 5).

Emotional control

The possibility of some people becoming depressed was mentioned earlier – they often lose their will to move. Others who have difficulty in making sense of their surroundings (see Chapter 6) may react to their frustration and fear by becoming aggressive or withdrawn. This behaviour has to be avoided if you are to persuade them to move. The subject of managing fear to promote movement is dealt with in Chapter 4.

Motivation

Most of us do not have to urge ourselves to move during the course of the day. We move about in order to carry out everyday activities and for leisure or pleasure purposes. Sometimes, however, we do not feel like doing anything and have to make an enormous effort to persuade ourselves to 'get up and go'. The people you are caring for often have no desire to move, so it is up to you to persuade or motivate them to do so. Chapter 7 looks at ways of doing this.

Perception

Even when their eyesight is normal for their age group, people with dementia may misinterpret features in their surroundings. The brain fails to process the information coming from their eyes. So it is possible for a chair-sized space between two chairs to be mistaken for a chair, with the result that the person sits down onto the floor. Any strong colour contrast on the floor or shiny threshold strip may be 'seen' as a step – and the person may lose his balance and fall when he takes an unnecessary step up. These occurrences are very distressing – Chapter 6 suggests how you can help people to move about with more confidence.

What else can affect mobility?

All people with dementia are unique individuals. The impairments caused by dementia are likely to affect each one in different ways. Therefore the mobility difficulties of each one also vary. Unless you step in to give help, the impairments just described can affect their mobility.

In addition to the effects already described that can affect mobility, there are other ways in which it can be affected:

- physical problems;
- management policies;
- personal factors.

Physical problems

People with dementia may also be suffering from a variety of conditions associated with ageing. The expression *multiple pathology* is used to indicate this. Many of these conditions affect mobility: for example, the pain and movement limitations of arthritis and osteoporosis (see Glossary); the shortness of breath or lack of energy resulting from heart and lung conditions; the pain and discomfort arising from circulatory diseases; and the problems associated with deteriorating eyesight.

Management policies

Mobility can be reduced very quickly if restraint is practised. Some examples of restraint include trays fixed in front of people when they are seated in chairs or wheelchairs; the use of harnesses; very low chairs; or the practice of 'fencing in' people for long periods behind tables. Too much medication has a similar effect.

The way you approach your work is very important. If you have received dementia-specific training, you will know that people with dementia must be treated with respect and courtesy. You also know how important it is to encourage them to remain active and to help them to make use of their remaining skills and abilities for as long as possible.

Personal factors

SEATING

The effects of unsuitable seating on mobility have already been mentioned. Everyone must be provided with a chair that suits their own height and size, so that it is as easy as possible to get up and to sit down.

The chair should also be of a design that allows care staff to get close enough to give help when it is needed.

CLOTHING

Shoes and slippers that do not give enough support to the feet do not help people to move, and may contribute to falls (see Chapter 9). Ill-fitting clothing can do the same; for example, a man may trip over trousers that trail on the floor because they are being worn without belt or braces or because they are too long. Clothing that does not belong to the wearer may also add to the unwillingness to move, because it is unfamiliar. Insecure incontinence pads and drainage bags that are not hidden can cause distress and so discourage mobility.

All these are some of the factors that can contribute to the onset of mobility problems in people with dementia. The task of maintaining as much mobility as possible might seem to be daunting, but the benefits of doing so are great. The costs of immobility in terms of personal suffering, both physical and psychological, are hard to calculate.

What are the benefits of maintaining mobility?

This section looks at how both people with dementia and their carers, as well as managers of residential and nursing homes, can benefit when mobility is maintained.

Benefits for the individual

People who maintain some ability to move about have the personal satisfaction of retaining a small amount of independence. The activity helps to meet their need for exercise, gives them an outlet for their energy and may reduce their sense of frustration. The exercise is beneficial for their general health: it maintains the strength of muscles and the ease of joint movement, and the increased activity of the heart and lungs improves the circulation. They are more likely to sleep at night rather than by day, the risk of thrombosis (see Glossary) is reduced, and pressure sores and contractures (see Glossary) are prevented. With increased muscle power, bladder control often improves and constipation becomes less of a problem.

Benefits for carers and care workers

You need to use less physical effort when you help people who are able to carry out part of the movement for themselves. The risk of physical injury should therefore be reduced. You can gain much personal satisfaction from successfully maintaining reasonable levels of mobility, and your morale is boosted.

Carers benefit from the improved sleep patterns of the people they are caring for by being able to enjoy a less interrupted night's sleep themselves. If the ability to manage stairs can be maintained, it will not be necessary to bring the bed downstairs – this avoids the need to reorganise the home (see Chapter 10, Mr Patel). And the maintenance of a reasonable level of mobility delays or reduces the need for special equipment, such as a hoist.

Benefits for managers of residential or nursing homes

Managers can share in the sense of pride enjoyed by their care staff who are successfully keeping residents as mobile as possible. The home gains a good reputation for its achievements, and the managers should find it easier to recruit *and* retain staff. There should be less long-term sickness due to injury and therefore a reduced risk of claims for compensation. Running costs of the home should also be reduced, because less specialised equipment is required, expensive dressings for pressure sores are not necessary and fewer incontinence aids are likely to be needed.

Disadvantages of maintaining mobility

People who remain mobile without assistance are free to move about or wander; they may also get lost or fall. You need to watch them carefully in order to prevent avoidable incidents. These 'wanderers' often interfere with other people's belongings and may contribute to accidents involving others whom they try to help.

Carers often find wandering one of the most difficult and worrying problems to manage (see Chapter 10). Some of them feel that it would be easier to care for their loved ones if they were bed- or chair-bound. While it is easy to sympathise with these views, professionals must be able to convince carers that the possible consequences of immobility could be even worse.

The surroundings in which care is given also affect the behaviour of people with dementia. So, if you are to maintain their mobility, you need to be working in a 'dementia-friendly' environment. The building needs to be carefully planned to provide safe space inside and outside, and the choice of floor coverings, furnishings and fittings requires special attention (see Chapter 6, and suggestions for Further reading on p 123). Provided careful thought is given, this need not be an expensive process.

Conclusion

We tend to take for granted our ability to move about. It is usually only when we are sick or injured that we realise how much the loss of mobility can affect our life-style. In such circumstances, most of us are able to find the professional help that we need, or to fight for what we consider to be our rights as citizens. People with dementia are also citizens and have the same rights as any others. In 1986 the King's Fund Centre in London published a document on this subject. *Living Well into Old Age: Applying principles of good practice to services for people with dementia* sets out five key principles:

- their value as humans;
- their varied needs;
- their rights as citizens;
- their individuality; and
- their right to appropriate support that does not exploit family and friends.

Because dementia robs people of the ability to demand services that meet their needs, it is up to us to act on their behalf.

The chapters that follow show that immobility does not have to be the expected and accepted consequence of dementia. The message is a positive one – it is possible to lessen the problems that accompany dementia. Therefore, the promotion or maintenance of some useful level of mobility is a realistic and achievable aim.

References

Department of Health (1995) *The Health of the Nation. Health and well-being: a guide for older people*. HMSO, Manchester

World Health Organization (1990) Draft of Chapter V, categories F00–F99, *Mental and behavioural disorders. Clinical descriptions and diagnostic guidelines.* WHO, Geneva (Geneva Division of Mental Health, CH-1211, Geneva 27, Switzerland)

King's Fund Centre (1986) *Living Well into Old Age: Applying principles of good practice to services for people with dementia*, King's Fund, London

2 Making Communication Easier

Communicating with people with dementia may not be easy, but it is essential if they are to be asked or persuaded to move. This chapter suggests ways that will help you to do this.

Communication

It is convenient to think of communication occurring in three stages:

1 the giving;
2 the receiving; and
3 the response.

When you are trying to persuade a person with dementia to move, you must give the request in a way that helps them to understand what you want; then your message has the best chance of being received and acted upon. If you are successful, the response will be in the form of a movement or action – a spoken reply is not necessary.

Communication is made up of *verbal* and *non-verbal* parts – some of it is spoken and some is not. When you speak, you automatically use both – they cannot be separated. What you say and how you say it make a big difference to the way people respond, so you need to know how to adapt or change your approach to suit their needs and to persuade them to move.

Ways of making your verbal communication more effective are described in this chapter; the ones for non-verbal communication, involving gestures and cues, are in the following chapter.

Variations in ability to move

People with dementia vary in how willing and able they are to move:

- There are those who want to move and do so; some of them seem to move with a purpose in mind, and others to move about aimlessly throughout the day. People who wander do not need to be motivated to move, but rather to be persuaded to remain comfortably at rest for at least part of the day.
- Then there are those, lacking in motivation, who are able to move if asked or persuaded to do so. Ways of talking to this group are discussed in detail in this chapter.
- Finally, there are those who always refuse and others with complex problems who might benefit from the special help of an occupational therapist or physiotherapist (see pp 88–91).

Making communication more effective

Impaired hearing makes it more difficult to communicate with people with dementia, so it is important to check whether the person has a hearing aid and, if so, that it is in working order. You will need to supervise its use carefully, because the person may forget to fit it, be unable to turn it on and off, may fiddle with the settings during the day or simply refuse to wear it. You should also make sure that other aids that help with communication, such as glasses and dentures, are also being worn and fit correctly.

The initial approach

Even when glasses and hearing aids are being worn, you need to approach people thoughtfully. Move towards them from the front so that you do not startle them; if you arrive from the side you may alarm them with your sudden appearance. Approach slowly with a welcoming smile, but do not get too close; they may feel threatened if you do.

Attract their attention by addressing them by name and making eye contact. Give them the opportunity to greet you, and then introduce yourself or remind them who you are. Remember to control your hands and keep any gestures small and well away from their face; hand movements may be misinterpreted.

Mr Cash (introduced to you on p viii) is day-dreaming in his chair. A nurse approaches him from the front and greets him gently, 'Good afternoon, Mr Cash'. She pauses and repeats her greeting more firmly to attract his attention, 'Hullo, Mr Cash'. She gives him time to reply and then tells him who she is: 'My name is Mary, Mary Rushworth'. She shows him the name badge on her sweater. 'I've something to tell you.' She needs to explain something to him, so it is better if she also sits down. She seats herself facing him but to his side. In this position they are both able to see each other but she is out of his reach if he tries to kick her.

If you are approaching to help someone to move, you need to stay on your feet ready for action.

Why communication can be difficult

There are several reasons why communicating with people with dementia can be difficult:

- poor memory;
- difficulty in finding the right words;
- difficulty in understanding;
- slow responses;
- difficulty in locating sounds.

These difficulties have to be lessened or overcome if you are to persuade someone to move. We will look at each of them in turn.

Poor memory

Memory may be extremely poor, so people have difficulty in remembering what they have been asked to do, or what they are doing. You need to repeat your request or instruction several times, patiently, in order to help them complete the task.

Difficulty in finding the right words

People who have difficulty in finding the right words have what is known as a *dysphasic-type* problem. Give them the chance to express themselves as well as they can, without stepping in too quickly to help them. Watch their facial expression and body-language; their face and body posture give valuable clues to what they are trying to say.

Difficulty in understanding

Many people with dementia find it hard to understand what they are being asked to do. This is another dysphasic-type problem. Once again, it is up to you to help them to understand by making use of the approaches and cues suggested in this and the next chapter.

Slow responses

Responses to your requests may be slow or very slow indeed. Remember that, before they can move, people with dementia have to understand what is being asked of them, then prepare for the requested movement and, finally, carry it out. All these processes take time. People who also have Parkinsonism (see Glossary) are likely to need even more time, because the condition slows down all their responses.

If you do not give people enough time, you may help them when they could in fact carry out the movement unaided. They then miss both the opportunity and the satisfaction of moving 'under their own steam', and you give yourself unnecessary work and may risk injury.

Difficulty in locating sounds

People with dementia often find it hard to decide where sounds are coming from; this can cause communication difficulties for them and for you. The problem can be lessened by making sure that you approach and speak to them from the front, as described earlier in the section dealing with the initial approach.

When you are beside a person to help him to move, it is impossible to speak face-to-face or maintain eye contact. You are, however, well placed to speak directly into his ear and to attract his attention by gently increasing the pressure of your support. If two of you are helping him, it is important that only one of you speaks. People with dementia find it difficult enough to make sense of one voice.

Bear in mind that, because people with dementia have difficulty in locating the source of sounds, a request given to one person may be acted on by another, who also hears it. You should be aware of this possibility because there is always a chance that the other person might try to get up and then fall.

Methods of communication

Words do not always have to be spoken; they can also be written.

Writing

A written message can sometimes be very helpful, especially if the person has hearing difficulties. They are best written in a large, clear round hand, rather than in block capitals.

Some people retain the ability to read until quite late in dementia, but may not understand the meaning of the words. For example, they may be able to read out loud a request to 'Stand up, please', but do not carry it out even though they are able to do so. It would be easy for you, but wrong, to jump to the conclusion that they were refusing to stand up.

Speaking

The voice is a powerful tool and can be used to great effect. You can vary its volume, tone and pitch to assist in the delivery of a request. Shouting does not help people to understand, but slow, clear diction does. Sometimes speaking more quietly will attract a person's attention better than speaking louder. This strategy loses its impact if you use it too often though, because its value lies in the element of surprise.

Hearing tends to deteriorate with age and there is likely to be some loss of ability to hear higher sounds. So if you have a high-pitched voice, try to lower its pitch when you are talking. It is worth experimenting to check the effect.

The Alzheimer's Disease Society point out in their booklet *Caring for the Person with Dementia* (Lay and Wood 1994) that people with dementia are particularly sensitive to tone of voice and body language. So pay attention to your tone of voice and learn to control it, because any signs of irritation or impatience are likely to be picked up.

Making the best use of verbal communication

Communication can be made easier by:

- experimenting with wording;
- making direct requests;
- giving 'positive' instructions;
- wording for automatic movement.

Experimenting with words and wording

Although words account for only a relatively small percentage of the meaning of speech, they are still important.

People with dementia are more likely to understand words and expressions that are familiar to them, so make an effort to search for an appropriate vocabulary. Experimenting with other words and wording can make a difference and may enable them to understand. Family carers can often provide you with information about the words and expressions that they were used to. Repetition is essential and you can afford to use the same words a couple of times; after that, though, you need to re-word what you are saying because endless repetition of the same words is not helpful.

Making direct requests

On most occasions you want people to carry out movements or actions without too much delay. So express your request simply and politely, in a *direct* way that makes it quite clear what you are asking them to do.

Mr Cash does not move out of his chair unless he is asked to do so. His nurses find that he responds well to requests such as, 'Mr Cash, stand up, please', or 'Mr Cash, I want you to stand up, please'. They need to repeat the request and to add a few words of persuasion, 'I'll help you', or 'I'm going to help you', to encourage him to rise. However, if a nurse approaches him and asks, 'Mr Cash, would you like to stand up, please?', he usually replies politely with a 'No, thank you'.

Unfortunately, this commonly used *indirect* way of asking someone to do something, with the request worded as a question, invites the possibility of a refusal. So Mr Cash responds to the question, 'Would you like to stand up?', rather than to the request, 'Stand up, please'. The refusal, 'No, thank you', gives the nurse a problem which she then has to overcome. She does not argue, but moves quietly away and leaves him for a minute or two. She then returns to try again and makes sure that this time she words the request in a direct way. She is taking advantage of his impaired short-term memory and hoping that he has forgotten about her first effort. It is, however, not unknown for the person to refuse again, 'You've asked me that before, and I said, "no".' So such occurrences are best avoided in the first place.

When it is convenient, the nurses give Mr Cash a choice: 'Mr Cash, would you like to go to bed now?', or, 'Mr Cash, would you like to sit in this chair?'. By offering him choices, they are giving him the opportunity to make decisions – this is important.

Giving 'positive' instructions

The following sequence of events may be a familiar one. You are helping someone to walk and he starts to sit down on an imaginary chair. Either he slowly and deliberately bends his hips and knees as if to sit down or he announces that he is going to sit down. 'Don't sit down, don't sit down', you snap out quickly – and he sits down. He almost certainly does not hear the 'don't' in your instruction and responds to the 'sit down'. In such a situation, an instruction that is worded positively rather than negatively, such as 'Stand up – stay standing' is much more likely to produce the result you want. This strategy requires practice because we are all so used to saying 'Don't do this' or 'Don't do that'.

WHY DO PEOPLE TRY TO SIT DOWN LIKE THIS?

There are several reasons why people might attempt to sit down inappropriately:

- The sitting down is triggered by the sight of a distant chair. If this seems to be the case, you can use a positively phrased request and encourage the person to stay upright.

- The distance to be walked is too long. The walk may need to be shortened, but the problem can often be solved by allowing one or more short rests on chairs placed conveniently along the way.
- They forget what they are doing. They need frequent reminders.
- Their concentration is upset by too much noise or movement; a noisy radio or television can be very distracting. The effect of what is going on around people with dementia is often under-estimated. Their surroundings must be appropriate to their needs if they are to do their best.

Wording for automatic responses

Before considering how wording can be used to encourage movement at an automatic rather than at a thought-out level, it is useful to look at the difference between the two.

AUTOMATIC AND THOUGHT-OUT MOVEMENT

Most of us are fortunate enough not to have to think how to carry out each movement that we make during the course of our daily lives. We move at an automatic level that is entirely spontaneous and quite unlike the efforts we have to make when learning new skills, such as those required for skipping, swimming or dancing, for example. However, once the sequence of the new movements or activities can be carried out smoothly, the need for conscious control involving thought and concentration gradually disappears. With practice, fluency develops and the new movements are available for use at an automatic level. This leaves us free to turn our attention to other matters or to carry out other tasks at the same time.

ENCOURAGING AUTOMATIC MOVEMENT

People with dementia should be encouraged to move at this *automatic* level. The tendency for some of them to try to carry out very basic movements, such as rising to standing, at a thought-out level, needs to be overcome, because it can cause unnecessary difficulties or even failure. Pain, fear, anxiety and uncertainty need your attention.

Pain People who find movement painful will carry it out in a careful manner – they try to avoid the pain. This avoidance, which is natural to all of us, results in movements at a thought-out level. People with dementia may be unable to explain that they are in pain, but you will notice if a movement that is normally carried out fairly easily suddenly becomes difficult. The flare-up of an arthritic joint or the after-effects of a minor fall are possible causes, but the source of the pain needs to be found so that action can be taken and pain relief provided (see also Chapters 4 and 7).

Fear   This subject is dealt with in Chapter 4.

Anxiety and uncertainty   People who are anxious about moving need plenty of reassurance and encouragement. Physical support given effectively (see Chapter 5) will help them to feel more secure and enable them to move more spontaneously. People who move with uncertainty because they have difficulty in understanding what you want them to do usually respond well to strategies aimed at encouraging movement at an automatic level. Some strategies are described below, and others can be found in Chapter 7.

What you can do to encourage automatic movement

- Keep requests clear and short.
- Suggest the ease of the task.
- Use goal-based requests.

Clear, short requests

Requests should be clear and simple so that people have the best opportunity of understanding. A simple request such as 'Mr Cash, stand up, please' is more likely to be understood and carried out at an automatic level than is a complicated one. For example, a long request, such as 'Mr Cash, I want you to use both your arms to push yourself up into standing' is almost certain to confuse him and usually leads to failure.

The ease of the task

This can be suggested by the wording you use and by the tone of your voice. So, for example, the words, 'Mr Cash, just stand up, please', expressed in a light, casual way convey the idea that this is going to be easy and that you expect him to succeed. Because people with dementia are particularly receptive to tone of voice and body language, they are able to pick up your unspoken message.

Goal-based requests

These can be very helpful in certain circumstances. Sometimes people fail to rise when asked to do so, even though they show that they have understood and you know that they are able to stand up. It is probable that they are trying to carry out the rising action at a thought-out level. If this seems to be the case, use a different approach: use wording that draws attention to a different task. 'Miss Kenny, there's a cup of tea for you on the table' is one example. Reaching the cup of tea is the *goal* – it involves Miss Kenny in *standing up*, as well as walking across the room to sit at the table, but is not mentioned.

People who seem to be having difficulty getting out of bed in the morning may also be attempting to move at a thought-out level. They may respond to a similar approach that avoids any mention of getting up, such as, 'Mrs Polanszky, I'll help you to dress – come and sit on this chair'. With a little imagination and thought, you can think of wording to suit many different situations.

Talking to people with dementia

This chapter has concentrated on the verbal strategies that you can use to promote mobility. There are other reasons why you will also want to talk to the people you are caring for. The ability of people with severe dementia to carry out a meaningful conversation may be very limited indeed. They should, however, be given the opportunity to do so and to be treated as if they do understand, even if you are almost certain that they do not. Some assistants make a habit of talking to others nearby and do not include the person they are caring for in the conversation. This is very poor practice and conveys a lack of respect.

There is a simple solution to the problem of finding topics to talk about if you run out of ideas. You can provide a running commentary while carrying out any task. For example, there are opportunities for describing the choice and fitting of shoes before walking; the rearrangement of cushions, pillows or rugs afterwards; and the final positioning of the person's walking aid for later use.

KEY POINTS

- Communication for movement *is* possible.
- Give more than enough time for a person to respond.
- Speak clearly and simply.
- Find words and expressions familiar to the individual.
- Use repetition generously.
- Use wording to encourage movement at an automatic level.
- Talk to people with dementia even if you are doubtful about their ability to understand.
- Make determined efforts to understand what they are trying to convey.

TRAINING EXERCISES

1 Imagine that you are a person with dementia who has someone at either side talking to him. Ask two colleagues to speak to you, one after the other, several times. How do you feel about it?

2 Practise wording useful instructions in a *direct* way with a colleague. Make a point of listening to other people's requests worded as a question in an *indirect* way and silently reword them in a *direct* way.

Reference

Lay, Chris and Wood, Bob (1994) *Caring for the Person with Dementia: A guide for families and other carers.* Alzheimer's Disease Society, London

3 Making the Most of Non-verbal Communication

In this chapter a variety of different gestures and cues are suggested. They help people with dementia to understand better the words that you are using. They also make it possible for you to persuade them to move in a particular direction. Movement strategies are discussed in the final section.

Non-verbal communication

Some experts think that the unspoken, non-verbal parts of communication are more important than the spoken ones: the figures quoted are 55 per cent non-verbal as opposed to 45 per cent verbal. The verbal percentage is made up of 7 per cent from the words themselves and 38 per cent from use of the voice (Argle 1975). It is therefore important that you make the very best use of non-verbal communication.

The initial approach to people with dementia was described in the previous chapter. Facial expression is particularly important because so much meaning and emotion can be shown by it. But the posture of your head and body and the gestures you make with your hands also play their part. A smiling approach with arms outstretched provides a non-threatening welcome, whereas the same smile accompanied by folded arms does not. You need to be aware of your own body language and to learn to read that of the people you are caring for; this improves with practice.

Using gestures and cues

There are many different gestures and cues that you can use to help people with dementia. The ones suggested in this chapter will help you with the task of promoting and maintaining their mobility. *Cues* are useful in many areas of dementia care; for example, laying out someone's clothes in a logical order gives cues that may make it possible for him to dress successfully without help. And the prompts given to a forgetful person during a conversation provide cues that help him to complete his sentences.

You need a range of cues that make it easier for people to understand which movement you want them to do, and in which direction.

Direction of movement

All movement involves a direction: for example, standing *up*, sitting *down*, moving *across/along/up*, leaning *forwards* or *backwards*. You may want the people you are caring for to carry out some of these movements during the course of the day when a basic change of position is needed. Of these, the words 'up' in 'Stand up, please' and 'down' in 'Sit down, please' do not present any problems, because 'stand' and 'sit' are usually enough to produce the right movement.

This is not the case with 'move' and 'lean', because neither of these words tells you or the person you are talking to anything about the direction of the movement. They need the addition of a word that indicates the direction, such as 'along', 'forwards' or 'backwards'. Although you now have enough information to decide about the direction of the move or the lean, the same does not always apply to people with dementia. The solution lies in using cues that encourage movement in a specific direction when you give your spoken request to move.

Making the most of movement cues

There are several different types that you can use:

- gestures;
- touch cues;
- visual cues;
- sound cues;
- goal-based cues/requests.

USING GESTURES

Gestures are a normal part of everyday speech and are used by everybody. You probably make them during a telephone conversation, even though they cannot be seen by the person at the other end of the line. Some gestures are very familiar: the high beckoning sweep of a raised arm and open hand that says, 'Come here, please'; the low wide arc of an upturned hand that offers someone a seat; and the little patting movements on the seat beside you that invite someone to 'Come and sit here'.

You can almost make your hands speak, but you do need to be careful how you use them; a friendly gesture made too close to someone's face may be viewed as threatening and provoke a hostile response. For your gesture to be effective, the person must be able to see it, so check that glasses are being worn if they are required. Then decide which gesture you are going to make and carry it out carefully.

With practice and by watching reactions, you can become skilled at making gestures to suit the varying needs of many different individuals. As some people do not like to be touched, gestures provide a very valuable means of communication.

USING TOUCH CUES

Touch cues are gestures that make physical contact. Touching needs to be done with care and sensitivity. You should certainly tell people you are caring for that you are going to touch them, so that they are not taken unawares (see Chapter 8 for more about using touch).

For transfers   When you want someone to swing his hips across during a transfer from one seat to another, give a series of gentle taps or nudges to his hips with the palm or fingers of your relaxed hand. This touch cue to the side of his buttocks shows him quite clearly in which direction to move.

To encourage standing up   Give a touch cue to the seated person's spine, between the shoulder blades. The cue makes clearer your request to 'Stand up, please'. Use a slight forwards and upwards pressure of the fingers of your hand to indicate the direction of the movement. Or, instead of the cue just described, sweep your hand firmly but gently up the person's upper back to provide a moving touch cue. Some people respond better to this moving cue than to the stationary one – it is up to you to watch their reactions and decide which of these cues is the more effective. Ways of using your hands effectively to give touch cues are explained in Chapter 8.

Where should you position yourself? In the interests of back care, you should always take up a good posture. You could stand facing the person, slightly to one side, but it is probably advisable for you to stand at his side so that you are both facing in the same direction. Stand with one foot one normal pace in front of the other, and bend your knees so that you do not need to stoop (Figure 1). In this position, known as *walk-standing*, you are able to give a touch cue with your hand near the person; if the need arises, you can also provide any help without reaching or losing your balance. The furniture should be arranged so that you have enough room to work from the side of the chair. Further guidance on how to position yourself while helping someone to rise can be found in Chapter 5.

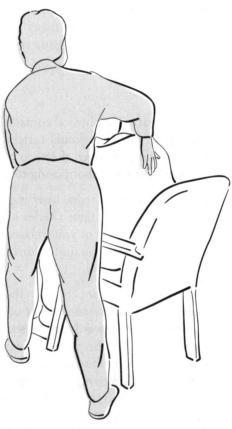

Figure 1   Giving a touch cue with the assistant in walk-standing at the person's side.

USING VISUAL CUES

Demonstrating a movement in front of the person is one way of providing a visual cue.

Moving back in a chair   The side-to-side rocking movement needed to move from the front to the back of a chair is a difficult one to explain to someone with dementia. You can try a gesture using the palms of your hands, to indicate the direction of the movement in the chair, when you ask him to 'Move back in your chair, please'. Another possibility, is to give a touch cue to his knees, with a slight backward pressure.

> **Miss Kenny** (introduced to you on p viii) has never responded to such a cue on its own, but does so when a demonstration is added. An assistant stands in front of Miss Kenny and tells her that she wants her to move back in her chair. Then, with her knees slightly bent, the assistant wiggles her hips from side to side, to demonstrate the way to move back in the chair. Finally, she repeats the request, 'Miss Kenny, move to the back of your chair, please', and adds a gesture to indicate the backwards direction. The demonstration usually makes Miss Kenny laugh and she moves back in her chair.

Many older people find it impossible to transfer their weight from one buttock to the other, but, like Miss Kenny, move backwards in their own way. They use a series of small movements: raising both hips from the chair and immediately lowering them, moving a few centimetres backwards each time until they reach the back.

Kerbs and steps   are often not well defined or easily seen, so there is often a real risk of older people tripping or landing heavily. This does not improve their confidence and can lead to a general reluctance to move.

You can provide a valuable visual cue by stepping up, or stepping down, just before the person moves. Give a warning at the same time, 'Here's a step'. The change in level of your head and body and the verbal warning are usually enough to make sure that he steps up or down safely. If you are giving physical help, he may also feel the change in the support that you are giving.

Stairs   If the step or steps are deep ones, such as stair-risers, it is difficult to move ahead of the person who needs assistance. Use a different strategy and place one foot onto the step above so that your bent forward knee acts as a visual cue. From this stable position, you can continue to give assistance and allow him to step up completely before doing so fully yourself. This method works well when going up a flight of stairs, but a different one is required for coming down them (see Chapter 4).

USING SOUND AS A CUE

Sounds can be used to attract someone's attention *and* to show him the direction of the movement you want. They can be particularly helpful for people with poor eyesight.

Transfers   You can encourage a chair-to-chair transfer by slapping the seat of the adjacent chair to produce a 'chair noise'. With the chairs positioned appropriately (see Chapter 5) so that the person can move across safely, give the sound cue at the same time as your request, 'Sit *here*, please' or 'Move into *this* chair'.

Lying down on a bed   Many people with dementia find it difficult to position themselves correctly along the length of a bed when they are asked to lie down: they usually finish up across its width instead. You can help with this problem by slapping the pillows at the head of the bed to make a 'pillow noise'. The sound gains the person's attention and shows him where the head of the bed is. You can use an additional cue by helping him to feel the pillows with one hand just before you ask him to lie down. The combination of these two cues is usually very effective.

USING A GOAL-BASED CUE/REQUEST

This type of cue can be used to encourage the leaning forwards movement that is the start of the standing up process.

Leaning forwards   When you ask someone who is seated to 'Put your nose over your toes', he is likely to lean forwards. If he raises his toes towards his nose instead, you can give a demonstration of the forward-leaning movement that is required. This adds to the original goal-based cue (see also Chapter 2).

OTHER CUES

Others cues can be found in Appendix 2, in the lists of strategies suggested for each activity. You can also invent others to suit the specific needs of individual people you are caring for.

Making the most of movement strategies

In addition to the range of cues described above, there are other strategies that you can use to encourage particular activities. *Movement strategies* can help you with the following activities:

- rising from a chair without arms;
- forward leaning in preparation for rising;
- assisted walking;
- sitting down.

Rising from a chair without arms

People usually find it easier to rise from a chair with arms than from one without. Pushing up into standing from the seat is difficult and it needs enough hip movement to allow the person to lean well forwards. Many older people have stiff hips, which make this difficult. The solution is to provide a substitute for the chair arms.

CREATING SUBSTITUTE CHAIR ARMS

The method described below uses two assistants, but it can easily be adapted for use by one. Start by positioning yourselves on either side of the person's chair, so that you are all facing in the same direction. Stand in the same walk-standing position, with your knees bent, that was suggested for giving touch cues to encourage rising (p 26). Your 'leading' thighs provide substitute chair arms that the person can push against (Figure 2). Chapter 5 looks at other ways of using substitute chair arms.

The point of contact on your thigh will vary with your stature and that of the person you are helping; he can use any part of the your mid-thigh, down to the knee, to push against.

Forward leaning in preparation for rising

People with dementia sometimes find it particularly difficult to lean forwards. It is an important movement because it is the first part of standing up. There are several different ways of overcoming the difficulty. You can either use the goal-based cue described above or a strategy that results in a forward lean. There are two ways of achieving this:

- providing substitute extensions to chair arms;
- using the back of a chair.

PROVIDING SUBSTITUTE EXTENSIONS TO CHAIR ARMS

You can use this method with any suitable chair, whether it has arms or not. Take up the position that creates substitute chair arms, as described on page 29, but stand a little further forward. In this way, you can provide a substitute extension to the arm of the person's chair. When he places his hands on your thigh, or is helped to do so, he is automatically brought away from the back of the chair into the leaning forwards position in readiness for standing up. This method is even more effective when there are two assistants (see Chapter 5).

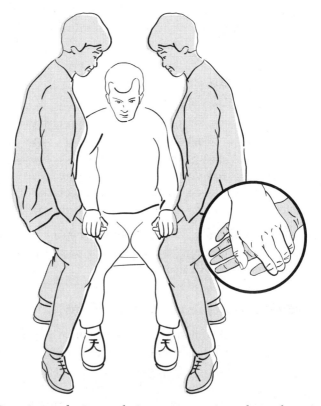

Figure 2   Creating substitute chair arms – using the palm-to-palm thumb hold against a firm pillar of support.

USING THE BACK OF A CHAIR

Place a stout dining-type chair a short distance in front of the person, so that the back of the chair faces him; if he uses a walking frame, that can be used instead. Then ask him to place one hand forwards onto the back of the chair or the frame (Figure 3). By providing him with something to reach for, you make sure that he finishes up in the forward leaning position. He may need a little time to get used to the new position, and to sitting without any support to his back, before he attempts the rising movement.

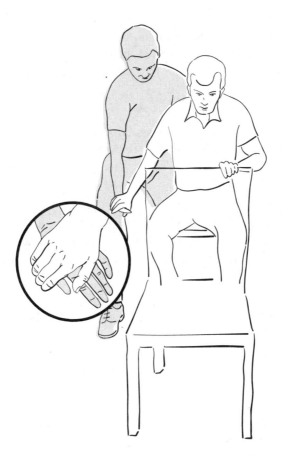

Figure 3   Using the back of a chair to encourage forward leaning, or to prevent 'gripping' when there is only one assistant.

Rising with one hand forward   The person is now sitting forwards ready to stand up, but he is only able to *push* himself up with one hand – the one that remains on the arm of the chair he is sitting in. He will manage to rise when he pushes himself up with this hand and *presses down* with his forward hand so that the chair or walking aid does not tip. However, if he tries to pull himself up on the back of the chair or walking aid with his forward hand, it will tip. If this happens, do not steady the chair/walking aid, but allow the tipping to take place. Then gently tell him that the chair is tipping because he is *pulling* on it. With your encouragement, he is able to turn the 'pull' into a 'press down'. He can then rise to standing.

Note   When the difficulty of leaning forwards has lessened, you can stop using this method. He should now be able to lean forwards and keep his hands on the chair arms in readiness for rising. Rising with *both* hands on the chair arms is what you are aiming for.

Assisted walking

There is a natural rhythm to walking. Space may be limited when you are helping someone to walk, so it is important to establish the rhythm quickly.

UNISON WALKING

A rhythm can be achieved almost immediately if you walk in step with the person you are helping – *unison walking*. Positioned at his side, in close physical contact, you are able to step forward at the same time that he does and with the same foot (Figure 4).

People with Parkinsonism   Unison walking makes it easier to maintain a good rhythm, so it is particularly useful for people with Parkinsonism who find this difficult. If the person's feet start 'stuttering' (see Glossary) with tiny quick steps up and down almost on the spot, pause for a moment or two and then restart the unison walking. If someone has difficulty in starting or restarting walking, either urge him to imagine climbing a step or give him a visual cue that encourages stepping – raise one of your knees in an exaggerated manner. Then step forward with him and walk in unison with him.

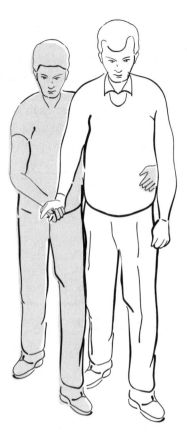

Figure 4   Unison walking: the assistant uses the palm-to-palm thumb hold and keeps the person's elbow straight.

Sitting down

Some people reach the chair uneventfully with or without help, but if they are positioned in the traditional, 'safe' manner with their back to it, they are reluctant to sit down. This seems to be because they cannot see the seat. The solution is therefore simple – position them side-on to the chair so that they can see it throughout the sitting down movement and allow them to move sideways onto it. You can always give some little directional taps to their hips to encourage a safe landing. Managing the process of sitting down with help is described in Chapter 5.

MANAGING A WALKING AID

Someone who is using a walking aid should be encouraged to approach the chair across its front. The pathway needs to be curved so that the walking aid does not get in the way. Figure 5 shows the position of the walking aid immediately before the person sits down – you can see that you need to encourage him to move the aid well beyond the far leg of the chair. He is then able to see the chair while he sits down on it.

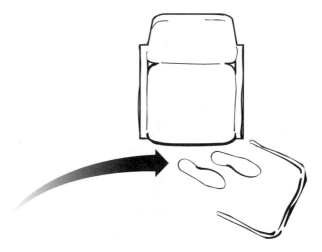

Figure 5   Position of the walking aid immediately before the person sits down.

Conclusion

You can experiment with the use of cues and invent others to suit the particular needs of the people you are caring for. The shape and nature of gestures are likely to vary from person to person, but be aware of the possibility of unconsciously causing offence with them: the meaning of a gesture in one culture may be different in another.

Reference

Argle, JA et al (1975) *Bodily Communication*. International Universities Press, New York

KEY POINTS

- A combination of verbal and non-verbal strategies can ease communication difficulties.
- Give 'cues' to show the person the direction of the movement required.
- Warn people before you touch them.
- Use your thigh as a substitute chair arm or as a substitute extension to a chair arm.
- Walk 'in unison' with people when you help them.
- Ensure that the person can see the chair throughout the sitting down sequence.

TRAINING EXERCISES

Work with two colleagues.

1 Experiment with gestures to indicate the direction of a movement; for example, *back* in a chair; *along* the edge of a bed; turn *over* in bed. Does your 'client' find the gestures helpful? Can they be misinterpreted?

2 Positioned carefully (back care), give a stationary, then a moving, touch cue to a seated colleague's upper back, to enhance your spoken request to stand up. Does your colleague find one more effective than the other? Change places with your colleague and repeat the exercise.

3 Compare the ease of rising from a chair without arms with that of rising with the aid of substitute chair arms. Change places so that each of you makes the comparison and practises creating a substitute chair arm.

4 Managing Fear

People with dementia may be afraid of moving and falling. Some of them refuse to move because of this fear but are able to tell you that they are afraid. Others are not able to put their fear into words but show it by their behaviour. This chapter takes a close look at some of the reasons for this fear and suggests ways to make movement less of an ordeal for people.

Recognising fear

When people with dementia are seated and you ask them to move, they may show that they are afraid by pressing themselves into their chairs. Some react more strongly: they push themselves backwards with their feet and grip tightly onto the chair arms. If they are lying down in bed when you approach them, they may clutch at the bed-clothes and become stiff and rigid. Whether the response is slight or more obvious, their body posture is saying, 'No, I don't want to move – I'm afraid'. They need a great deal of reassurance from you, in addition to the use of strategies to help them to overcome or minimise their fear. The strategies are described later in this chapter.

Understanding the reasons for fear

Some reasons why older people might be afraid to move are:

- previous falls;
- pain;
- difficulty in adjusting to changes of position;
- difficulty in making sense of their surroundings.

It is worth remembering that, although they seem to be refusing to move, it is possible that they do not understand what you want them to do. Alternatively, they may be trying to carry out the movement at a thought-out level rather than at an automatic one (see Chapter 3). Some say, 'No', but do not mean it; however, with experience you learn to tell the difference between a 'No' that means 'Yes', and one that really means 'No'.

Previous falls

Some people refuse to stand or walk because they have fallen in the past. They may, understandably, be afraid of falling again or they may not trust their legs to support them any more.

Pain

It is easy to understand that people who are in pain may not want to move. But how are you to know who is in pain and who is not? The simple answer is that some people can tell you and others cannot. Those who are able to do so can explain that they do not want to move because they are in pain. Those who cannot, depend on others to recognise that they are in pain from the way that they are behaving.

SEVERE PAIN

Generally speaking, it is not difficult for you to recognise those who are in severe pain; their distress shows in the expression on their faces and their body posture. These people are likely to need some form of pain relief prescribed by a doctor.

MILD PAIN

Mild pain, also known as low-grade pain, is often very difficult to detect. However, the people you are caring for may give you some idea where the pain is by their behaviour: they may show signs of distress when one of their limbs is moved, they may avoid moving as usual or they may be reluctant to take weight on one of their legs. You should report what you have seen, because the site and cause of any pain need to be found, so that any necessary treatment can be given.

POSSIBLE CAUSES

A fracture may be discovered some time after a fall that had seemed insignificant. Many older people, especially women, suffer from osteoporosis; this causes a loss of bone density and makes their bones particularly liable to fracture. Osteoporosis may also be the cause of the pain.

FEELING PAIN

Unfortunately, some care workers ignore these signals of pain, and dismiss them as 'attention-seeking'. Some even believe that people with dementia do not feel pain. This may be true in a few cases but, nevertheless, it is important to treat each one as an individual with feelings, and with emotions.

Treatment

The management of pain will vary according to its cause, but it is likely to include some suitable medication. Other possibilities are discussed in Chapter 7 (p 70).

Difficulty in adjusting to changes of position

For some people with dementia, the fear of moving seems to be caused by their difficulty in adjusting to changes in position. When they are sitting or lying down, they feel stable and secure; they are well supported by the back of the chair or the mattress and they have become familiar with what they can see around them. A change of position upsets this feeling of security and a short period of confusion and uncertainty follows. It takes several seconds for them to become used to the sights and sensations of the new position – this is why it is so important not to hurry them.

Difficulty in making sense of their surroundings

People who have difficulty in making sense of their immediate surroundings must be faced with a very confusing world – one filled with meaningless sights and sounds. So it is not surprising if they are anxious and reluctant or afraid to move about in it. You need to be aware of the possible causes of this and to do your best to make the environment a more friendly place. This subject is dealt with more fully in Chapter 6.

Activities that can cause fear

Some people with dementia find the following movements frightening and may refuse to carry them out:

- rising from lying down to sitting on the edge of the bed;
- going down steps or stairs;
- rising from sitting.

You can lessen their fears by offering them plenty of physical and psychological support. Some simple strategies that you can use during these movements are described below.

Rising from lying to sitting on the edge of the bed

This activity involves major changes of position: an initial move from lying flat (supine) to lying on one side, followed by a complex one that finishes in the sitting position on the edge of the bed. This second one involves movement of the head and body from the horizontal to the vertical position. During this change there are moments of great instability; the bed supports the whole length of the body at the start of the movement and only the buttocks at the end. People become disorientated by these changes of position, and are understandably afraid of falling off the bed. Seeing the drop to the floor from a low bed, 45cm (18 inches) from the top of the mattress, is alarming enough, but from a hospital bed it is worse. These are usually kept higher so that they conform to health and safety legislation aimed at reducing back injuries among staff.

WHAT YOU CAN DO

First of all, you can prevent the person from seeing the floor during this change of position by using a *gap-filling strategy*, and then you can give plenty of reassurance while he moves. The staff at a nursing home were able to make use of this strategy to overcome the unexplained 'aggressive' behaviour of a new resident. How they set about it is described below.

Finding out the cause of 'aggressive' behaviour

Mrs Polanszky (introduced to you on p ix was transferred to a nursing home because the small residential home was unable to cope with her increasingly aggressive behaviour. She had been lashing out at the care assistants – none of whom spoke Polish – when they tried to help her to move. The nursing home started to assess her and to record how often she became aggressive. Anna, an experienced Polish staff nurse, spent some time with her. She confirmed that Mrs Polanszky was not responding to English but recognised and spoke occasional words in garbled Polish. She had repeated the word 'fall' several times. It seemed possible that she was hitting out because of a fear of falling. The recording of the 'aggressive' behaviour showed that it happened most often when she was being helped out of bed – this can be a frightening experience.

Reducing the fear of getting out of bed

Anna helped Mrs Polanszky to get out of bed the next day. She spoke to her reassuringly in Polish, and made sure that she blocked the view of the drop to the floor while helping her out of bed. First of all, she placed a pillow lengthways on the edge of the bed, at the level of Mrs Polanszky's head and on the side to which she was going to turn. She then helped Mrs Polanszky to lie with her knees bent up, so that it was impossible for her to roll off the bed. Anna positioned herself between Mrs Polanszky's shoulders and hips so that she could both assist and block the view of the floor with her own body. Finally, she carried out the whole sequence slowly and smoothly, reassuring Mrs Polanszky and giving her plenty of time to adjust to each change of position. There was no aggressive response. Anna included the strategy in Mrs Polanszky's care plan and taught the English-speaking nurses to say 'You are safe' in Polish, so that they could reassure her.

Going down stairs

Many fit people feel insecure when they go down a flight of stairs. If they are wearing bifocal spectacles or carrying a very precious load, they are likely to hesitate at the top and descend slowly, taking a great deal of care. Others avoid stepping onto an empty downward-moving escalator – they wait until there is somebody in front of them. So it is not surprising if some people with dementia show signs of insecurity and a fear of falling when they are asked to go down stairs. A well-lit stairway and a solid handrail are of course essential for safety reasons, but they do not necessarily overcome people's reluctance to step down into the apparently empty space.

WHAT YOU CAN DO

You can partially block the sight of the unpleasant descent of the stairs if you step down just before the person you are helping does so. When you position yourself safely, slightly in front of him, you are able to observe him and give help; he must of course use the handrail for support. When there are two assistants, one of you can completely block the view of the stairs by going down in front of him while the other helps at his side. Both of these are *gap-filling strategies*.

An alternative solution

Mr Patel (introduced to you on p viii) needs to be able to manage the stairs. Mrs Patel is anxious that her husband should sleep in his own bed, in his own room, as long as possible. The staircase in their terraced house is very steep and narrow, and there is only one handrail. So Mrs Patel is worried about her husband's safety when he comes downstairs facing forwards in the normal way. She prefers to get him to hold onto the handrail with both hands. In this position he is able to step sideways down one stair at a time by placing one foot on the tread and bringing the second one to join it. Mrs Patel helps from a safe position behind him; there is room for two people sideways on. She uses a special handling belt round her husband's waist to give her something to hold onto, because she knows that it is not safe to hold onto his clothing. The belt makes her feel much more confident during the descent, and Mr Patel feels more secure.

Although Mrs Patel chose this particular method for safety reasons, there is no reason why it should not be used as a gap-filling strategy for someone who is frightened of going downstairs. If this had been the case with Mr Patel, this method would have provided a way of preventing him from seeing the alarming descent ahead – he has to face the wall in order to hold onto the handrail.

Rising from sitting to standing

This is an important activity. The ability to stand up gives you the opportunity to walk away from your chair; it is a vital part of the standing up, walking and sitting down sequence. It is also a very complex activity, involving leaning far enough forwards to make it possible for you to raise your hips off the chair seat and put your weight onto your feet. During the leaning forwards movement, you have to move your head and shoulders well beyond your feet before you are able to raise your hips off the chair seat.

It is not difficult to understand why some people are reluctant to stand up; it is because they have to lean so far forwards into the empty space ahead. Some may refuse to try. Those who are afraid show their fear by holding onto the chair arms and pressing themselves into their chair.

WHAT YOU CAN DO TO ENCOURAGE LEANING FORWARDS

You can lessen the fear of leaning forwards before standing up simply by putting something in front of the person – a *gap-filler*. The most convenient object is likely to be a dining chair; there is usually one available. By placing the chair in front of him you achieve three things: first, you fill the alarming empty space ahead; second, you give him something to hold onto once he has risen; and third, you make him feel safer.

Choosing a suitable gap-filler The chair you choose should be strong and solid; a dining chair or a small easy chair is usually suitable. It needs to be stable, easy to move in and out of position and with a back that is not too high. If the person has a walking aid, you can try using that instead of the chair, but its fragile-looking structure may not provide enough reassurance.

Positioning the gap-filler Place the chair with its back towards the person. It is important that you position it carefully, because it is not safe to allow him to haul himself up by means of the chair back. The correct position is likely to be about 30cm (12 inches) in front of his feet. This distance will vary with the length of his arms; if they are short, it will be less. The chair back provides support for him once he has stood up.

It is often possible to stop using this gap-filling strategy after a period of time. As their fear lessens or is overcome, you may find that people are happy to rise when their walking aid, instead of the chair, is placed in front of them. Others improve so much that they do not need anything in front of them at all.

Gripping chair arms

You will find that some people with dementia have a tendency to grip their chair arms when asked to stand up – they are showing you that they are afraid. They may even attempt to rise while continuing to hold onto their chair. This can be prevented with the use of the palm-to-palm thumb hold. The hold is described in detail in the next chapter (p 54).

Conclusion

Some people with dementia may be afraid to move, but there is much that you can do to overcome or lessen their fears. You can reassure them with the words that you use and with the help that you give. You can also put into practice the strategies that have been suggested in this chapter. The next four chapters describe other ways of increasing the chances of moving successfully.

KEY POINTS

- Listen to what the people you are caring for are telling you.
- Watch their behaviour when you ask them to move.
- Discover why they are afraid to move.
- Find the source of any pain and get treatment started.
- Use gap-filling strategies to lessen their fears.
- Give them time to adjust to changes of position.
- Reassure with words and give help effectively.

TRAINING EXERCISES

1 Sit down and close your eyes. Imagine that you are in the mountains, sitting on a big rock on the edge of a vertical drop or rocky gorge. You are asked to stand up – first with nothing at all in front of you and then with a good solid stone wall in front of you. How did you feel? Did you stand up?

2 Lie down flat on a single bed. First of all, roll slowly onto your side and think about the drop to the floor. Compare that experience with this one: roll towards a colleague who is standing close beside the bed, so that you cannot see the drop to the floor. Which one makes you feel safer?

5 Making Assistance More Effective

People with dementia need to stay as mobile as possible, for as long as possible. They are likely to need more help as the dementia progresses. Many of them manage to move when you are there to give them instructions and to boost their confidence. Others need your physical help. This chapter looks at ways of making this assistance as effective as possible.

Moving and handling

Legislation

The present legislation aims to protect the safety of workers and sets out the responsibilities of employers and employees:

- Under the Health and Safety at Work Act etc 1974 (HSW Act), employers and employees have a 'duty of care' towards each other (see Glossary). Employers must provide training and a safe place of work, and employees are expected to be responsible for their own safety and for that of their fellow workers.
- The Manual Handling Operations Regulations 1992 added to the duties placed on employers and others by the HSW Act. They introduced an ergonomic approach (see Glossary) to assessing the risk of injury before carrying out activities where manual handling cannot be avoided. The Regulations apply to the manual handling of people as well as of objects.

REASONS FOR THE 1992 LEGISLATION

The HSW Act was designed to reduce injuries in the workplace, but the rising number of accidents showed that the legislation was not being effective. By 1990, 1.5 million working days were being lost every year in the National Health Service. Many nurses were sustaining back injuries as a direct result of handling patients, and the cost to the health service was enormous.

WHAT DO THE 1992 REGULATIONS SAY?

They say that employers should:

- *avoid*, wherever possible, involving employees in manual handling that involves a risk;
- *assess* the risks if manual handling cannot be avoided; and
- *reduce* the risks to the lowest level that is reasonably practicable.

The Royal College of Nursing (RCN) backs a 'no lifting' policy but does not rule out manual assistance when the risk of injury is low. This means that hoists and other aids should be used for people who cannot move 'under their own steam', because the risk of injury is high. When manual assistance is used to help people to move, it should be effective (see p 49) and the level of (low) risk kept under constant review.

TO WHOM DO THE REGULATIONS APPLY?

The Regulations are an extension of the 1974 HSW Act and as such apply to all employers whose employees handle loads (see Glossary). So they affect nursing and residential homes, day hospitals and day centres just as much as hospitals.

HOW ARE THE RISKS ASSESSED?

The risks are assessed under four main headings:

- the task;
- the load;
- the environment;
- the capabilities of the individual.

An assessment carried out by the nurses caring for Miss Kenny (introduced to you on p viii) shows what questions they asked to establish the level of risk.

Miss Kenny was walking with the help of one nurse until she suffered a small stroke (see p 51). After a couple of days she was feeling better, and the nurses were anxious to get her moving again. The hoist was being used to lift her out of bed into a chair, but she was managing to transfer safely from the chair to a commode and was able to stand to a support for a few moments, with extra help from two nurses. So was it safe to help her walk a few steps?

That, then, was the *task*. Miss Kenny would need effective manual assistance – would this involve twisting, stooping, reaching or any unusual posture? No, it would not. Would her legs collapse? This was possible, but they knew that she could stand to a support and take most of her weight.

Next the *load*: how much does she weigh? They knew that – she is weighed regularly, and it is recorded on her personal file. She is neither big nor stout, her medical condition has not changed and she co-operates with them. Would they be able to hold her securely? Their hands might slide on her clothing, so a handling belt would be safer and would increase their confidence as well as Miss Kenny's.

What about the *environment*? Is there enough space in her room? It is fairly small but they could use the corridor, which does not slope and is wide enough to allow the three of them to walk side by side very comfortably. They would need to make a last-minute check – just before they set out – that there was nothing hazardous on the corridor floor that they might trip over.

Their *individual capabilities:* both nurses are fit, healthy, strong and not suffering from over-tiredness. One is mature and very experienced and the other young and recently qualified. They both receive regular updates to their basic moving and handling training, and are very aware of the responsibility they have for each other's safety. They work well together.

What did they decide?   They agreed that there was some risk to themselves if they tried to be too ambitious. So they decided to reduce the risk to a minimum by keeping the first walk very short and by arranging for a third nurse to follow them with a wheelchair. Miss Kenny would wear her shoes with a broad heel so that she would have a good stable base to walk on. They agreed that, to improve communication with her, only one of them would give the instructions or encouragement (see Chapter 2).

The questions you should ask will obviously vary with the circumstances. Some assessments are much more complicated and detailed than this one and are recorded on special forms.

Guidance for professional workers

In addition to this national legislation, professional carers should follow any guidance issued by their professional body. You can find details of some useful publications at the end of this chapter.

Guidance for carers

Carers are not covered by any such legislation and may be giving physical help to their relative, neighbour or friend without the benefit of any advice or training. Many devoted carers provide 24-hour care for seven days a week, which is physically and mentally exhausting. Fatigue is known to contribute to injuries, so such carers are very much at risk. If you have to give physical help, it is important to get advice on how best to do so safely; your GP may be able to refer you to a physiotherapist or occupational therapist for this.

Training for professional carers

You need to be physically fit and trained to move and handle people using suitable techniques. The training sessions should combine theory and practice, and be appropriate to your type of work. You need to be able to assess the risks and to use the equipment and aids that are provided for you, as well as being competent to move and handle people. The training and revision sessions you attend should always be led by suitably qualified instructors.

INFORMATION ON MOVING AND HANDLING TECHNIQUES

This book is not a manual of moving and handling techniques; there are reference books devoted to the subject. Particularly useful are *The Guide* to *Handling of Patients* (Royal College of Nursing 1997) and *A Manual of Handling People: A health and safety guide for carers* (Tuohy-Main 1994). Both these books contain much valuable information on manual handling techniques and the assessment of risks.

Giving effective assistance

You need to boost the confidence of the people you are caring for while you help them to move. The hints and strategies described below should make your help and support more effective:

- using an appropriate position;
- overcoming gripping of chair arms;
- providing a firm pillar of support;
- grading assistance.

Using an appropriate position

You must position yourself carefully when you are preparing to give physical help to someone. Your starting position is very important – it can affect the outcome of the movement you are attempting. If you are observing the principles of good back care and are well positioned, you should be able to give the smooth, fuss-free physical help that is needed. You are then more likely to be trusted by the people you are helping, who will respond more positively and move with greater confidence.

POSITION FOR RISING TO STANDING

Take up the walk-standing position, at the side of the person, as if you are about to give a touch cue to promote rising (see Chapter 3). Your hips and knees should be bent (Figure 6). This position provides you with the stable base that you need for giving help. It is absolutely essential that you get *as close as possible* to him if you are to maintain a good posture and give effective help. The thickness of the sides of his chair or any other design features must not prevent you from getting close. A large fully upholstered easy chair with wide arms and well-padded sides is not suitable (see Chapter 9 on how to obtain advice on seating).

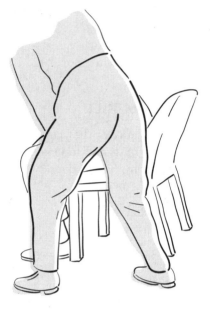

Figure 6   Walk-standing position, showing bent knees and hips.

Helping a client to rise

Mr Cash needs help to rise from his chair. His nurse tells him that she would like him to stand up. She gently helps him to place his hands on the chair arms and places her 'outer' hand lightly over one of his – the one close to her. She passes her 'inner' hand behind his back and places it flat over his far hip, so that she will be able to help him effectively. Then she tells him that he is going to rise, 'Mr Cash, you're going to stand up. Ready, stand *up*'. She helps him to raise his hips off the chair and removes her 'outer' hand from over his when he is ready to release it from the chair arm. She immediately offers her 'outer' hand to him, palm upwards, so that she can support his hand in the palm-to-palm thumb hold (see pp 53–54) while he completes the rising movement.

The nurse could have supported Mr Cash's elbow instead of his hip, or she could have used a handling belt round his waist (see how to obtain special equipment in Chapter 9).

POSITION FOR APPROACHING A CHAIR

Some people with dementia misjudge the distance between themselves and the chair they are approaching. Those who are anxious almost throw themselves at it; they either just manage to land on its edge or they badly misjudge the distance and risk landing on the floor. When you are supporting someone, or merely walking beside him, you can encourage him to make a more controlled approach – this is important because falls need to be prevented (see 'Falls' on p 101). It is, however, difficult to make sure that people who move about without help are safe when you are not there.

When there is one assistant When you are giving physical assistance on your own, you need to plan ahead and use positive instructions (see Chapter 2). Position yourself at the person's side. Plan to approach the chair, slightly to its side, so that he is nearest to it; he must be able to keep it in his sight and reach for the far chair arm with his free hand. Tell him in a firm but reassuring tone of voice, to 'Keep walking, keep walking', and be ready, if necessary, to guide his hips onto the chair seat. You can do this by moving slightly behind him and using your thigh and knee to nudge or slide his hips sideways onto the chair.

When there are two assistants

Miss Kenny has been managing to approach a chair and to sit in it, with one assistant, until recently. She had a small stroke a few days ago and now needs the support of two people to help her reach a chair.

The two assistants have to alter the way they approach the chair, so that the one nearest to it does not prevent Miss Kenny from getting close enough to sit on it. If, when they try to get close, they walk across its front, they finish up with Miss Kenny's back to the chair – she is then reluctant to sit down because she cannot see it. They find that they can get her closer if the assistant nearest to it steps to the side of the chair when they reach it. From that position slightly behind Miss Kenny, this assistant is able to help her to place her hand on the far arm of the chair and to swing her hips onto the seat. The other assistant supports Miss Kenny throughout as usual.

POSITION FOR TRANSFERS WHEN THERE IS ONE ASSISTANT

If you are the only person available to help someone to carry out a chair-to-chair or similar transfer, you need to position yourself very carefully. As well as giving any cues that might be required, you need to be able to help him to reach for the far arm of the receiving chair and to guide his hips onto the chair. With the chairs correctly placed, approximately at right angles to each other, the space *behind and between* them offers you the best position (Figure 7). From here, you are able to control and assist the transfer, as well as maintaining a good posture; if you try to help at his side, you will not be able to assist or control the transfer in the same way.

You may need to use the *gap-filling strategy* (described in Chapter 4) of placing a chair in the space in front of your client, to make sure that the transfer is successful. The addition of this chair reassures him and boosts his confidence. It also helps people with stiff hips who are not able to reach far enough across to the other chair. They need to stand up first and hold onto the back of the gap-filling chair, before sitting down on the receiving chair.

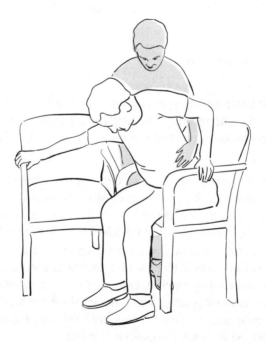

Figure 7   Position for assisting a chair-to-chair transfer.

When there are two assistants When two assistants are available, one can be positioned at the person's side. This assistant gives the instructions and the cues. The second assistant positions herself in the space behind and between the chairs. It is important not to confuse the person you are helping, so this assistant does not give any spoken instructions but helps him to position his hand on the far chair arm and swing his hips across onto the receiving chair. Both assistants are able to maintain a good posture throughout.

Note The help you give during any transfer should not involve a huge effort; an 'assist' must not become a 'lift'.

Overcoming gripping of chair arms

Some people with dementia who are afraid or unwilling to move tend to cling protectively onto the arms of their chair – this was mentioned in the previous chapter. They fail to release their hands from the chair arms and try to stand up while still gripping onto them; they may even succeed in partially lifting the chair off the floor. The person who is helping him may not be aware of what is happening and suddenly feels an enormous increase in the weight as the load of the chair is added. The resulting jerk can be unpleasant and puzzling, and may cause a back injury.

You can overcome this problem by taking the person's hand in your own *before* he puts his hands on the chair arms in readiness for standing up. You can then place the back of *your* hand against the chair arm, making it impossible for him to grip it – your hand separates his from the arm of the chair. The *palm-to-palm thumb hold* is ideal for this purpose. Just follow the steps outlined in the paragraph 'Taking up the palm-to-palm thumb hold' below. If, however, the person has already gripped the chair arms, you will need to release his hands before you help him to rise.

RELEASING THE PERSON'S HAND FROM THE CHAIR ARM

The way to release a person's hands from the chair arm in order to take up the palm-to-palm thumb hold is described in Chapter 8 (p 84).

TAKING UP THE PALM-TO-PALM THUMB HOLD

If you are on the person's right side, you offer your right hand, with the palm upwards, to his downward-facing right hand. You take his hand, curling your thumb around his and wrapping your fingers over the back of his hand (Figure 8).

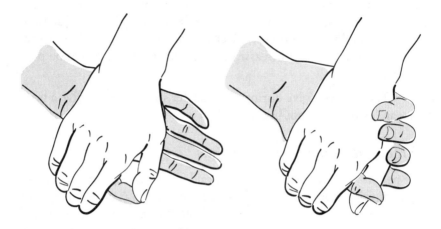

Figure 8   The palm-to-palm thumb hold, showing the assistant's left hand (palm up) supporting the person's left hand (palm down).

USING THE PALM-TO-PALM THUMB HOLD

With two assistants   If there are two of you assisting, both of his hands can be separated from the arms of his chair by means of the palm-to-palm thumb hold.

With one assistant   If you are alone, he can still make rising impossible by gripping onto the chair arm with his other hand. This must be prevented, so before helping him to rise, place this hand on the back of a chair that you have positioned in front of him (see Figure 3). Make sure that he presses down with this hand (see 'Using the back of a chair' in Chapter 3).

Providing a firm pillar of support

Most older people who are having difficulty in rising to standing make use of their arms to add to the power provided by their hip and thigh muscles. They usually push against something: for example, the arms of the chair, if they are not too high; the seat of the chair, if there are no arms; the edge of the bed; nearby furniture; or even their own thighs. It is likely that you will have to encourage them to use their arms.

A FIRM PILLAR OF SUPPORT DURING RISING TO STANDING

You should make sure that there is something solid for the person to push against:

- chair arms or
- substitute chair arms.

Using chair arms   Tell him that you would like him to stand up. Then gently encourage him to place his hands on the arms of his chair. He can now use the chair arms as a *firm pillar of support* to push against. If, however, you are using the palm-to-palm thumb hold (described opposite), you can place the back of your own hand against the chair arm so that he is still pushing against a solid support but your hand is in between it and his hand.

Using substitute chair arms   If you are using the palm-to-palm thumb hold and his chair has wooden arms, they make it too uncomfortable for the back of your hand. In this case, you can make a substitute chair arm with your thigh or knee to provide the firm pillar of support (see Chapter 3 on how to create substitute chair arms).

Note   Both these methods that use the palm-to-palm thumb hold *and* the firm pillar of support allow you to give effective assistance to the person's hands for rising *and* to continue giving it during walking, without making any changes in the support.

A FIRM PILLAR OF SUPPORT DURING RISING FROM A BED EDGE

Rising from the edge of a bed is particularly difficult. The mattress is soft and the bed is often too low – and it becomes even lower when the person compresses the mattress while he pushes against it with his hands.

Using two assistants   If you are working with a colleague, you can seat yourselves close on either side of the person to make substitute chair arms with your thighs – you should all have your feet firmly on the floor. These substitute chair arms raise the level of the surface and provide the person with a firm pillar of support to push against.

Using one assistant   If you are the only assistant, you can position a chair with arms, or a stool, against the bed on one side of the person and seat yourself on the other. In this way, you provide him with a firm pillar of support on both sides.

Grading assistance

You should always encourage people to contribute as much effort as they can to every movement they attempt. You can then top up their efforts by giving them some assistance. The help you give may have to be graded, or varied, during a movement, but should *never* amount to a lift.

DURING RISING TO STANDING

Many people require more help at the beginning of the rising to standing sequence than at the end of it. If you do not grade your assistance, you run the risk of giving more than is needed, and you may as a result decide that they are less able than they in fact are.

'Propping' When you give someone more help than he needs, he may lean heavily on you. If this 'propping' does occur, you must gradually reduce the amount of support you are giving. You should then feel him starting to take more or all of his own body weight.

Allowing people to push effectively During the rising movement, you should always allow the person to finish pushing against the support, *before* he removes his hands from it and rises into the standing position. At the end of the push, his elbows should be as *straight* as possible and he should be at the point of transferring his weight onto his feet.

Unfortunately, some well-intentioned care staff move the person's hands away from the chair arms, or other support, before he is ready to transfer his weight onto his feet. By doing this, they make it impossible for him to push when he needs to and he feels very insecure.

Making walking as easy as possible

Helping people to walk is not always easy. You need to be sure that you can give the most effective support and deal with any problems that might occur by:

- avoiding changes of support;
- using an effective method;
- using a walking aid;
- preventing 'grabbing'.

Avoiding changes of support

It is important to avoid any unnecessary changes of support while you are helping someone to walk. Continuity gives him confidence and increases his trust in you. You can continue using the same support for rising and for walking (see the 'Note' on p 55). When you use the palm-to-palm thumb hold and support him behind his back, or under his elbow and forearm, you are able to walk 'in unison' with him (p 32).

Using an effective method of support

Some people tend to bend their elbow while you help them to walk. If you possibly can, keep the person's arm straight and support it against your body (see Figure 4) – it is then much easier for you to give effective assistance. Encourage him to push down into your supporting hand – this helps him to keep his elbow straight. This downward push, or thrust, in a 'walking stick position' makes the introduction of a walking aid much easier, because the same downward thrust is needed.

TOWING

The practice of some assistants to walk backwards while holding both of the person's hands is totally unacceptable; it is unnatural and extremely dangerous. Towing an older person at arm's length with one hand, like a child, is demeaning. You should walk in unison with people who require assistance, and offer a crooked arm to those who do not need support but who like to walk in a friendly fashion, arm in arm.

BACKWARD LEANING

Some people who need help to rise, lean backwards when they are standing up and preparing to walk. Sometimes the backward leaning disappears as soon as they start walking, but often it does not. Even if you ask them to 'Stand up straight' or to 'Lean forwards', they seem to be unable to correct their abnormal posture. Pulling them upright is not the answer; in fact it makes matters worse, because they lean even further back. If someone is inclined to lean backwards when he walks, obtain the advice of a physiotherapist. **Warning:** if the leaning is very extreme, do not even attempt walking; it could be dangerous.

Preventing grabbing

If you are the only person helping someone to walk, you will be supporting one of his hands and the other one will be free. He may therefore use this hand to grab at furniture, door frames or people. This tendency needs to be overcome, because it interrupts the normal rhythm of walking and is very dangerous.

OCCUPYING THE FREE HAND

Mr Patel has recently started to grab at the door frames while his wife is helping him to walk. This is making it very difficult for her to manage him at home. She tells Mark, the community psychiatric nurse, that she is becoming increasingly worried, because it now takes her so much longer to get him from one room to another. Mark feels that a recent minor fall has probably increased her husband's anxiety.

Holding a handkerchief

They discuss possible solutions and decide that Mrs Patel needs to reassure him and to try giving him a handkerchief to hold in one hand when she helps him to walk. At the next visit, Mrs Patel is much more cheerful, and feels that the handkerchief has helped to reduce the grabbing. On a couple of occasions, she needed to hold both of his hands; she did this by making a small alteration in the way she was supporting him. She also discovered that she can occupy his free hand in other ways, by getting her husband to carry different objects, such as a book or a rolled newspaper.

The suggestion made by the community psychiatric nurse was helpful. Mrs Patel was quick to use her ingenuity and found alternatives for the problem.

Using a walking aid

If a person's ability to walk improves and he needs less support from you, it is possible that he might manage with a walking aid. So seek the advice of a physiotherapist or an occupational therapist, who will assess his abilities and provide a suitable aid of the right height if one is appropriate. A walking frame with wheels that have a *built-in braking system* is the most commonly used piece of equipment; it can be pushed along to provide constant support. The subject of walking aids is covered in more detail in Chapter 9.

Preventing personal injury

Although it is the responsibility of your employer to provide you with a safe working environment, you have a responsibility for not putting yourself or others at risk. You must follow any local as well as national guidance on good practice as well as using your common sense.

Any strategies and approaches that lessen the amount of assistance needed should reduce your risk of being injured; many have been suggested in this chapter and in Chapters 2, 3 and 4.

Preventing injury to hands

It can be very painful to have your hand squeezed hard. If you offer someone your whole hand, including the fingers, to hold onto to, you make it possible for him to inadvertently squash your fingers. The pain of deliberate or accidental squeezing may force you to withdraw your hand from the hold. If this occurs while you are helping him to walk, it might result in a fall. Accidental squeezing may occur as a result of a gripping reflex, which can happen when you place the whole of your hand into his. The use of the *palm-to-palm thumb hold* avoids this, but still provides the support of a whole hand. This is because, although the palms of your hands are in contact, only the two thumbs are linked and the fingers are free (see Figure 8 on p 54).

The palm-to-palm thumb hold is suitable for use with most people and prevents them from damaging your hands. Even a determined effort to hurt you is unlikely to succeed, because of the relatively small diameter of your thumb. It is also easy and painless to wriggle your thumb free when you have finished helping the person.

Conclusion

Working with people with dementia is always demanding. It requires a great deal of mental and physical energy. People who do not have any problems with mobility are still likely to need your help to get from one point to another: you have to persuade them to move, and to accompany and guide them. Those who find moving difficult make even bigger demands on your physical energy. They depend on your ability to help them to move. The main physical effort must come from them, though, so it is up to you to encourage them to move with the least possible help. You can increase the effectiveness of your assistance by using the strategies described in this and the previous chapters.

KEY POINTS

- Giving effective assistance is more than a physical act; it is a skill that requires understanding, thought and sensitivity.
- Your basic training in moving and handling should be thorough and regularly refreshed.
- Maintain a good posture while you work.
- Encourage people to move 'under their own power'.
- Help them enough to enable them to complete the movement.
- Make your physical support as effective as possible.
- Regularly review the abilities of the people you are caring for.
- Be responsible for the safety of your own body.
- Don't be afraid to seek help and advice, especially of a physiotherapist.

TRAINING EXERCISES

Rising to standing.

1 Experience the 'feel' of pushing against a firm pillar of support on both sides: (a) using the chair arms, and (b) using substitute chair arms created from the thighs of two colleagues who offer you some help. Then, experience pushing up into standing with your hands supported in your colleagues' hands (do not use the chair arms or substitute chair arms, just use the support offered by their hands).

2 Repeat exercise 1 and decide which methods make you, as a 'client', feel most confident.

3 Repeat exercise 1 as an assistant and decide which positions help you to be most effective.

References

Royal College of Nursing (1997) *The Guide to the Handling of Patients,* 4th edn. The National Back Pain Association in collaboration with the Royal College of Nursing, London

Tuohy-Main, K (1994) *A Manual of Handling People: A health and safety guide for carers.* Connie Brown, Tucson AZ (2990 East Greenlee Street, Tucson AZ 85716, USA)

RELEVANT PUBLICATIONS

L21 *Management of Health and Safety at Work Regulations 1992 – Approved Code of Practice.* HSE Books, Sudbury (PO Box 1999, Sudbury, CO10 6FS)

L23 *Manual handling – Guidance on Regulations. Manual Handling Operations Regulations* (1992). HSE Books, Sudbury (PO Box 1999, Sudbury, CO10 6FS)

Royal College of Nursing (1996) *Code of Practice for Patient Handling.* RCN, London

Royal College of Nursing (1996) *Introducing a Safer Patient Handling Policy.* RCN, London

Royal College of Nursing (1996) *Manual Handling Assessment in Hospitals and the Community.* RCN, London

Tullett S (1996) *Health and Safety in Care Homes: A practical guide.* Age Concern Books, London

6 The Environment

People with dementia often lose the ability to make sense of their surroundings. They tend to misinterpret ordinary familiar sights and sounds, and as a result become confused and afraid. This can affect their willingness to move. You need to try to understand the reasons for their reactions and to help them to move with more confidence in their surroundings.

Interpreting the environment

Most of us take for granted our ability to make sense of small changes in our familiar home environment; people with dementia depend on us to do this for them. We can help them by using an empathetic approach – 'putting ourselves in their shoes' – by reassuring them about features in their surroundings that might confuse or frighten them, or cause a fall.

Home surroundings and their effect

Interior surroundings make a big impact on people with dementia who are able to walk from one room to another, with or without your help. Any changes in their surroundings caused by lighting, sunlight and noise, and features such as doorways and changes in the texture of floor coverings can confuse them and interrupt the rhythm of their walking. The misinterpretation of some sights and sounds can lead to a fall. The following examples show how this can happen.

- Someone mistakes the chair-sized space, separating two armchairs positioned side by side, for a chair, and sits down on the floor.

• One person is asked to move to an adjacent chair. Another person, mistakenly thinking that the request is aimed at him, moves and risks a fall.

It is likely that both these examples occurred as a direct result of dementia, because the information received from the eyes and ears was not processed accurately by the person's brain. In addition, the information is not likely to have been of the highest quality, because of impaired eyesight and hearing.

Changeable features that can affect mobility

People with dementia seem to have as much difficulty in making sense of familiar features as of unfamiliar ones. They are often confused by the effects of artificial lighting and sunlight, which they may misinterpret, and can become distressed and agitated by noise.

ARTIFICIAL LIGHTING AND SUNLIGHT

No one can be certain how people with dementia interpret changes in their surroundings caused by strong lighting or sunlight, but it would not be unreasonable to guess that they mistake dark shadows for holes or steps and patches of sunlight for water. People who are able to walk unaided tend to step over dark shadows that look like steps, and walk round or avoid the ones that they interpret as holes. They also avoid the patches of sunlight that they probably mistake for water. Whilst both actions interrupt the flow of walking, it is the stepping action that upsets their balance and risks causing a fall.

How do people with dementia interpret a dazzling dust-laden shaft of sunlight that crosses a room, or the very distinct shadow of a window on the floor? These are particularly puzzling and can easily bring someone to a halt.

All these incidents with artificial lighting or sunlight can very easily be prevented by altering the position of lamps and by partially drawing blinds and curtains.

NOISE

A constant noise from a radio or television is not necessary. Continuous and over-loud noises can upset people and make communication very difficult. Your voice has to struggle against this background, making it impossible for you to use any strategies that depend on the loudness or tone of your voice suggested in Chapter 2. You also need to bear in mind that the people you are caring for are unlikely to be able to put their distress into words and that many of them cannot move away from the noise to a more peaceful area without help. They may, as a result, become more agitated and less able to concentrate, making it extremely difficult for you to gain their co-operation when you want them to move.

Permanent features that can affect mobility

The planning of nursing and residential homes and hospital facilities for people with dementia requires a great deal of experience and specialised knowledge. Even a specially designed layout can be far from ideal for the purposes of mobility. For example, corridors are not wide enough to allow three people – a person with two assistants – to walk side by side, let alone to pass someone in a wheelchair; lounges are so cramped that walking aids cannot be left beside their users; and colour schemes are followed so rigidly that armchairs 'disappear' into matching carpets and curtains. Space in a private house or flat may be even more limited, with narrow hallways and small rooms filled with furniture that can make moving about very difficult.

Note   The details of several booklets on designing buildings for people with dementia are given in the 'Further reading'.

There are many other features in a normal domestic, institutional or private care setting that can be confusing for people with dementia and which upset the flow and rhythm of walking:

- shiny threshold strips;
- strong colour contrast of flooring;
- highly polished floor;
- changes in texture of floor covering;
- uneven floors;
- doorways.

SHINY THRESHOLD STRIPS

Some people may react to a shiny threshold strip in the same way as to a single step, by 'stepping' over it. So, unless you reassure them that the floor is flat, they lift one foot up and land heavily. They experience the same unpleasant sensation that you feel when you step down a bottom stair that is not there.

This *stepping* action is distressing for them, so make sure, as far as possible, that it does not happen. A few simple words such as 'The floor is flat – the floor is flat' spoken in a calm even manner is usually enough. The reassuring tone of your voice is likely to be more effective than the words you use.

There are of course people who are able to walk unaided, and who also tend to misinterpret the strips as steps. They cannot be warned unless a care worker happens to be close at the time – they may lose their balance and risk falling as a result of stepping. It is usually possible, however, to prevent the problem by arranging for the strips to be painted to match the floor covering, so that they are not so noticeable.

STRONG COLOUR CONTRAST OF FLOORING

Any sharp change of colour where different floor coverings meet, any well-defined patterns on vinyl-type flooring or jazzy designs on carpets may also cause stepping. And some zig-zag patterns can actually make the whole floor look uneven, an impression that understandably discourages walking. Flower or leaf designs woven into a carpet may attract the attention of people with dementia who are walking about; they risk falling when they stoop down to pick up the flowers or leaves.

There is no quick solution to the problems caused by the patterned floor coverings just described, unless you can move the people to a different area. The permanent solution is obviously to replace the floor coverings as soon as possible. Plain short-pile carpets, with a waterproof finish, and textured sheeting, that meet each other with a gentle colour contrast, should be chosen. These provide the best surface for people to walk on.

HIGHLY POLISHED FLOORS

Polished floors are more likely to be found in hospital corridors, wards and departments than in a domestic or nursing and residential home setting. Such floors are usually non-slip, but are seen as being wet and slippery by most older people, including those with dementia. Their reluctance to walk on what they see as an unsafe surface is reasonable and understandable – it is also impossible to explain to someone with dementia that the floor is not actually slippery, although it looks as if it is.

All wooden and other hard surface floors need to suit the special needs of the people using them. The use of non-slip dressings is not the answer unless it produces a matt, or a semi-matt, finish – a non-slip surface that shines does not solve the problem. You and your colleagues may have to insist that the shine is removed.

CHANGES IN TEXTURE OF FLOOR COVERINGS

You take for granted the change in sensation of walking from a hard surface onto a soft carpet – you do not even hesitate. Your brain immediately processes the sensations received through your feet and you know that you are walking on a carpet; it feels different but it is a familiar sensation. People with dementia are not so fortunate because their brain either fails or is slow to process the sensations. It is up to you to reassure them with your calm manner and tone of voice. Tell them that 'The floor is hard – the floor is hard – the floor is soft – the floor is soft', while you maintain the rhythm of walking.

UNEVEN FLOORS

Some floors are not entirely level. There may be slight humps and hollows that nobody can see. When you walk over them, you immediately 'feel' them with your feet and accept them, but people with dementia do not. You may therefore need to reassure them after you have both walked over these unseen little defects. Or, if you can remember where they are, you can warn individuals what to expect.

SLOPES

Some people treat steeply sloping corridors as if they were level; they fail to change the way they walk to suit the slope. Help by telling them that it is an 'uphill' or 'downhill' slope. In this way you are able to maintain their rhythm of walking on a slope.

DOORWAYS

People with dementia often hesitate or stop when they pass through a doorway. Sometimes there is a threshold strip across the entrance, which adds to their uncertainty, but the hesitation can happen when there is no strip. We cannot be sure, but it seems likely that while they are inside the doorway, the light in their peripheral vision (see Glossary) is temporarily cut off; this loss of light from both sides confuses them and they tend to stop. In order to prevent the hesitation and maintain the rhythm of their walking, reassure them and tell them that you are passing through a doorway.

Light to dark Doors do not always lead from one well-lit area to another well-lit one, which would be ideal, but may connect a light room with a dark corridor. If this is the case, remember to switch on the lights in the corridor before helping someone to walk through the doorway.

The contrast between light and dark can be even greater when entering or leaving a building. Imagine for a moment how you feel when you step outside into bright natural light or sunlight, from a dark interior. Dazzled by the light, you are forced to stop so that you can adjust to the brightness of the light. So give the people you are helping plenty of time and reassure them.

Conclusion

Our surroundings provide us with an endless source of stimulation and interest. Lighting, colour, furnishings, temperature and noise all affect us, as do other people's actions, activities and movements. But, unlike people with dementia, we are usually able to make sense of what is happening. For them, there are many features that may be confusing or a cause of fear. These affect their willingness to move about.

So watch their reactions and reassure them when they need it – not all of them misinterpret their surroundings. You also have to bear in mind that they may sometimes prefer you to remain silent; the physical support you are giving them may provide all the reassurance they need.

This chapter has looked at the features that are most likely to confuse people with dementia. It is possible to avoid some of them and to reduce the effects of others. Your role as an 'interpreter' is a valuable one. With your help, they may be able to move about in their surroundings with more confidence.

KEY POINTS

- People's surroundings can affect their willingness to move about.
- Some people misinterpret or become confused by features in their surroundings.
- Watch people's reactions and try to understand the reason for them.
- Deal with poor lighting, bright sunlight and noise.
- Expect some floor coverings, floors and doorways to upset the rhythm of walking.
- Act as an interpreter and tell the person you are helping what is there.
- Be reassuring and empathetic.

TRAINING EXERCISES

1 Look carefully at your own living area. What changes would be needed to make it suitable for people with dementia who misinterpret their surroundings?

2 Look at your present workplace with a colleague:

a Can you pick out any features that could confuse people with dementia? What changes could you make for their benefit?

b If it were to be upgraded or a new one planned, what mistakes in design could you warn against or prevent?

7 Planning for Success

This chapter suggests what you can do to make sure that people you are helping are given the best chance of succeeding. You need to be well motivated and to be interested in finding ways of easing their problems.

Increasing the chances of success

In addition to the strategies, approaches and ideas described in Chapters 2 to 6 there are other ways of making success more likely:

- lessening/avoiding fear and pain;
- preventing aggression/refusals;
- making movement enjoyable;
- encouraging automatic movement;
- setting realistic goals;
- using appropriate aids/equipment/furniture.

Lessening the effects of fear and pain

LESSENING FEAR

If you and your team use the gap-filling strategies described in Chapter 4, give help effectively (see Chapter 5) and use your voice to reassure the people you are helping, they should be able to move with more confidence. Your calm and controlled approach also makes the successful outcome of the movement more likely.

DEALING WITH PAIN

Any pain must of course be dealt with, whether it is mild or severe; otherwise a person may refuse to move (see pp 37–38). The possibility of giving heat treatment from a hot water bottle, hot pack or heat lamp should be considered with great caution because there is a high risk of burns. People with dementia are not able to tell the difference between a safe and an unsafe level of heat, and, like other older people, may have poor blood circulation.

Giving physiotherapy It is possible that a physiotherapist might consider using heat as a treatment after thoroughly assessing the person and his particular needs. She might, on the other hand, advise that an ice pack or a local ice cube massage around a painful joint is more suitable, or that the use of TENS (Transcutaneous Electrical Neuromuscular Stimulation) or acupressure might be helpful.

Using movement Apart from medication, a simple but safe way of providing some pain relief can be gained from the use of a rocking chair. The repetitive movement has a soothing effect and stimulates the body to produce a pain-relieving substance called endorphin. However, people with dementia are not likely to sit and rock unaided; you will need to give them frequent reminders, if not constant help, to keep the chair rocking.

Warning The rocking chair should be a comfortable, strongly built model that is designed and manufactured to a high standard. It is important to check that there is no possibility of it tipping up, especially while the person is being seated, and during its use.

Preventing aggression/refusal

Watch people's reactions carefully while you are working with them, so that you are aware of the effect that you as a person, your words and your actions are having on them.

WORDING YOUR REQUESTS CAREFULLY

The possibility of accidentally making it easy for them to refuse by the way you word your request was discussed in Chapter 2. So, avoid *asking* them whether they would like to move and politely *tell* them that they are going to do so. They may still refuse, but this is less likely. It is, of course, very important that you offer them choices, but to offer a choice when there is none available is not sensible.

If you are upsetting someone in some way or if he misunderstands what you are doing, stop immediately; an aggressive person is unlikely to carry out the movement you want. On some occasions, an apology may be all that is required: 'I'm sorry, Mr Cash, I didn't mean to upset you'; on others it may be necessary to politely leave him and try again later.

SHOWING UNDERSTANDING

People who are usually co-operative do not suddenly become aggressive without a reason. It is, nevertheless, not always easy to find an explanation for their unexpected behaviour. Bear in mind that they may have been upset by somebody else; have only just woken up from a deep sleep; be in pain; or be reacting to new or changed medication. There is also the possibility that you are, as far as they are concerned, interrupting their intention to carry out an important activity from their younger days. If you think that this last is the case, spend a few minutes talking to them about it. Then, when they are calmer, you can try repeating your request for the particular activity or movement that you need.

Making movement enjoyable

Getting to know more about the background and interests of each person helps you to know what they enjoy doing and what you can choose to motivate them. The choices are often:

- favourite interests and pastimes;
- music and movement;
- simple group games and activities.

USING FAVOURITE INTERESTS OR PASTIMES

Giving someone the opportunity to enjoy his favourite interest or pastime is one way of promoting activity that might not otherwise occur. He may leave his chair willingly and move to another room or area in order to spend time looking at family or other photographs, or he may find pleasure from walking with you outside or through a garden. There are many such activities that you can use to motivate people to move so long as they enjoy doing them.

Daily activities You can also make routine daily activities, such as going to the toilet, more attractive to reluctant individuals. Give them your undivided attention during these activities and talk to them while you are helping them – you can give a running commentary about what you are doing.

USING MUSIC

Music is important to most of us. Many people are happy to join in with a 'music and movement' group session, but refuse when exercises alone are suggested.

Miss Kenny is not interested when exercises are suggested, 'My exercise days are over', she says firmly. But she shows obvious enjoyment when she listens to well-chosen, familiar tunes that she remembers from her past. The beat of the music invites movement, so it is not long before she starts clapping her hands and tapping her feet with the others – and she joins in with the singing as well.

Other simple movements can be added to the clapping and the tapping to suit the abilities of the group. A sequence of different movements that can be repeated several times is what is needed – it is not a good idea to spend too long on one exercise or on one part of the body. By repeating the exercises several times, enough muscle and joint work can be given without causing too much fatigue or loss of concentration.

Training   Unless you have been trained to give exercises or movement to music, you should not start to do so until you have sought the advice of a physiotherapist or an occupational therapist. The therapist is able to advise you which people are suitable for the group. She may also help you with it until you know the routine and become confident enough to lead it.

Music therapists   Some hospitals are fortunate enough to be able to offer the services of a music therapist. These people are in very short supply, because they have to be trained musicians before they undergo training as therapists. They are, as a result, highly skilled in using music, singing and musical instruments in an imaginative way to encourage movement in the people they treat.

USING SIMPLE GAMES AND ACTIVITIES

Using music is not the only way to encourage movement. You can achieve some surprising results with simple games and activities when you use small pieces of colourful apparatus with people who are seated. For example, those who are normally afraid or reluctant to lean forwards may do so when they try to bounce foam balls into a container or while tossing small coloured beanbags into matching coloured hoops. It is essential that the games and activities are simple but not childish, and that there is an opportunity for laughter.

Length of exercise sessions   These do not need to be long; 15–20 minutes may be enough for people who have difficulty in concentrating. The sessions, however short, should always be well planned and they must achieve their agreed aims.

Safety precautions   It is essential that all those who lead groups, or who act as assistants, understand the reasons for any safety precautions *and* carry them out. One example might be to agree the maximum number of people that one assistant should be asked to supervise in a group. It is good practice to include such safety precautions in a written policy. Group leaders must also make sure that their assistants are well briefed and aware of anyone in the group who might need special attention.

Encouraging automatic responses

You will remember that people with dementia are more likely to succeed if they carry out movements or tasks at an automatic level rather than at a thought-out one (see p 19). In addition to these communication strategies there are a couple of new points for you to consider:

- use the least possible number of assistants;
- keep corrections to a minimum.

NUMBER OF ASSISTANTS

Some individuals are able to rise to standing when there is one assistant but fail to do so when there are two. This sounds curious, but the arrival of two assistants seems to suggest to these people that you expect the task to be difficult. As a result they struggle to carry it out at a thought-out level and fail. The arrival of only one assistant probably makes them think that it will be easy and they succeed.

KEEPING CORRECTIONS TO A MINIMUM

When you correct people, this tends to draw attention to the task and makes them think about it. If you must make corrections for safety reasons, carry them out slowly, in a very calm and reassuring manner. It is important to bear in mind that it is better for someone to succeed while using a somewhat strange but safe pattern of movement (see Glossary) than to fail because you insist that it be perfect. For example, people who sit with their legs crossed need to uncross them before standing up. Many do this quite automatically as they lean forwards, before their hips start to leave the chair seat. A correction is therefore not needed and would, if you made it, interrupt the movement unnecessarily.

Setting realistic goals

You can claim success for both of you when someone achieves a goal. So when you set a goal, involve the individual as much as possible, and make sure that the goal is realistic and attainable. Goals can be either short-term or long-term.

SHORT-TERM GOALS

These are usually part of a long-term goal, as a single step or a series of steps in it. You aim to achieve each step in a short period of time, such as days or weeks. Miss Kenny provides us with an example of a short-term goal with one step.

Miss Kenny had previously managed to move about without support, although she had needed someone to guide her from one place to another. Following a small stroke (see Chapter 5), however, she started to need the support of two people. After discussions with the physiotherapist, the nurses agreed that they should gradually reduce this level of help to one person. The nurses talked to Miss Kenny about this, and planned to achieve it in three weeks. They recorded the goal.

In less than three weeks, Miss Kenny was managing to move with the support of only one nurse. A successful outcome.

LONG-TERM GOALS

A long-term goal is one that you expect to work towards over a long period of time – months or years. You usually plan to achieve your long-term goals in stages by setting one or more short-term goals, as just described. Miss Kenny's nurses are now working towards a long-term maintenance goal, and so is Mrs Patel.

A relatively mobile client

> **Mr Patel** is visited regularly by Mark, a community psychiatric nurse. You will remember that Mrs Patel is anxious for her husband to continue sleeping upstairs for as long as possible, but their house has steep stairs (see Chapter 4). Mark agrees that this is a realistic aim and records in the care plan a goal to maintain Mr Patel's ability to manage stairs. He adds the words 'for the next three months', which reminds him to review the long-term goal.

A humble long-term goal   A long-term goal for people whose mobility is very limited might be to maintain their ability to stand to a support for one minute. There are benefits in achieving even this humble goal. It:

- eases nursing and dressing;
- relieves pressure on the client's buttocks and spine;
- stretches soft tissues;
- takes joints through their full available range;
- provides a source of exercise.

Note   Goals should be realistic, achievable, recorded and regularly reviewed.

Using appropriate aids and equipment

You are likely to need advice about many of the aids that are now available for sale or hire (see Chapter 9); a detailed assessment may be required before a suitable choice can be made. The right aid can solve a particular problem or make it possible for someone to carry out a task or activity with greater ease and confidence. The following example illustrates these points.

> **Mr Cash** is experiencing increasing difficulty in rising from a standard chair, and requires much more assistance than usual to achieve it. He is tall and his posture is poor. The nurses are anxious to keep him mobile, so they seek the advice of their physiotherapist. She assesses him and, with the agreement of the nursing team, arranges for the Red Cross to supply a chair of the correct height. The chair supports him in a good position, and makes rising much easier.

Conclusion

You need to approach the task of promoting mobility in a positive way. You must also be realistic. Goal-setting is helpful because it allows you and your colleagues to work with the same purpose in mind and to measure success. A regular review of the goals is, however, essential so that they can be altered if necessary. You need to remind yourself that dementia is a progressive condition and that people's abilities are likely to deteriorate over a period of time. This fact should not be used as a reason or excuse for not attempting to maintain mobility at the highest possible level, because the consequences of its loss for the individuals themselves, for care staff and for management are great. (The benefits of maintaining mobility were considered in detail in Chapter 1.)

We are all motivated to a great extent by success and by the satisfaction of doing a job well. Job satisfaction is increased when the whole team is working happily to agreed aims, and when the views and opinions of all grades of staff are valued. An effective leader makes sure that staff receive praise as well as guidance. Members of the team need to appreciate the different skills of fellow team members and support staff.

KEY POINTS

- Care staff should have a positive attitude and be well motivated.
- Use a co-ordinated team approach.
- Plan for success.
- Set realistic goals.
- Make movement enjoyable.
- Be sympathetic to individuals' problems.

TRAINING EXERCISES

Work with a group of your colleagues.

Select half a dozen of the people you are caring for and list their interests and pastimes.

a What facilities and opportunities for activities are you able to offer them at present?

b What other imaginative opportunities could you create, with the minimum of expense, to match their interests?

8 Making the Most of Touch

Touch provides you with ways of conveying messages silently; it is sometimes better than speaking. You are likely to think of your hands when touch is mentioned, but you can use other parts of your body as well. This chapter looks at how you can use touch to benefit the people you are caring for.

Hands

Hands can be used in many different ways: they can grip strongly, hold delicately, support safely, feel textures and shapes, and, when used for gestures or for touching, they can almost talk. For most gestures and for touching purposes, you are likely to be using your hands.

For touching, it is particularly important that you should be able to use your hands effectively. Soft, relaxed hands are kinder and more comfortable in use than hard, stiff ones. You may have to learn how to relax yours and to become familiar with the special feel of having them relaxed. A little practice is probably needed.

Learning to relax your hands

Start by sitting down, and place your hands, palms down, on your thighs; your elbows are at your sides and your hands are supported on your thighs. Now, keeping the 'heels' of your hands in contact with your thighs, gently stretch your fingers and thumbs, making them as straight as possible. Stretch for just a second and then stop, letting the fingers and thumbs fall back onto your thighs – all you have to do is to stop stretching, nothing else. Do this a couple of times until you can 'switch off' the stretch easily. Next, stand up and, with your arms hanging at your sides

– the palms of your hands will be facing inwards – practise the stretch-and-stop-stretching routine a couple of times as before.

When you have finished, notice the curved shape of your relaxed hands and fingers. Feel one relaxed hand with the other, and notice how soft and pliable it is. Note that if you pull the fingers out straight, they always return to the same curved position when you stop. Close your eyes and think about the softness and lack of effort in your relaxed hands. From time to time during the next few days, practise the little stretch-and-stop-stretching routine until you are able to relax your hands.

LEARNING MORE ABOUT RELAXATION

The stretch-and-stop-stretching routine is part of the Physiological Method of Relaxation described in the book *Simple Relaxation* (Mitchell 1977). It is a very effective physical method that is easy to learn. Because you use less energy when you carry out a physical activity in a relaxed manner, it is worth spending time learning how to relax the whole of your body. Then you will be able to relax when lying down, when seated, when standing and finally when active.

A brief version that you can use during the course of your daily work is given in Appendix 1. This little routine can help you to keep at least part of your body relaxed and your mind calm.

Using touch

Touching other people has to be done with care and sensitivity. Some people do not like to be touched and may object very strongly to it. It is also possible that they misinterpret the touching and think that you are assaulting them. This is why your initial approach, as described in Chapter 2, is so important. So always give them plenty of time and explain in simple terms what you are going to do. This is not easy when someone has difficulty in understanding what you are saying, but remind yourself that words are only one part of communication; your body language and posture, gestures, the expression on your face and tone of voice can also convey messages (see Chapter 2). Always watch people's reactions and be prepared to change your approach if necessary. And remember to tell your colleagues about any strategies that worked particularly well.

Using touch for different purposes

Touch can be used for a variety of different helpful purposes:

- for movement cues;
- while giving physical support;
- for silent communication;
- to relax or calm;
- to release a grip.

USING TOUCH FOR MOVEMENT CUES

Chapter 3 dealt with the use of gestures to improve communication and to show the direction of a movement. Touch cues made with your hands were also considered in the same chapter.

USING YOUR HANDS FOR TOUCH CUES

If you are going to make the best use of touch, you must be certain that you can do it in a way that is both comfortable and effective. For example, during a chair-to-chair transfer, or when someone approaches a chair to sit down, you may wish to give a series of little taps or nudges on the individual's hips to encourage turning. Practise giving and receiving this touch cue with a colleague, making sure that it feels friendly – and not like a poke. Use the soft inner surface of your fingers, or the palm of your open hand, starting lightly and then giving the taps or pats more firmly. Notice the difference between using a stiffened hand and a more relaxed one.

Improving your touch   Now do some revision of the very useful touch cue that encourages rising to standing. With a colleague, practise using your relaxed hand for the stationary cue and then for the moving one. For the stationary cue, place your fingers between your 'model's' shoulder blades – your fingers should be pointing down your model's spine towards the chair. To give the cue, use the soft pads of your fingers to press gently, but firmly, in a slightly upward and forward direction. For the moving cue, start lower down on your model's upper back, the fingers of your relaxed hand pointing downwards as before. Then sweep your hand gently, but firmly, up the spine with a slightly forward pressure. Finally, be the model yourself so that you can feel how your colleague uses her hands.

Using your body for touch cues

There is one occasion when you can use your body to provide a touch cue for communication purposes. This is when you want someone to move along the edge of the bed while he remains seated. Making a 'move along' gesture with your hands in line with the edge of the bed may be enough to help some people to understand what is required of them, but not for all. So try moving into the individual's personal space instead, as described in the example below.

Mrs Polanszky's ability to understand English varies from day to day. The nursing staff need to use a variety of cues to help her. She is a well-built woman and needs as much exercise as possible during her daily routine. Moving along the edge of the bed, in a series of little sideways movements, is one of the exercises written into her care plan. It is carried out routinely each time that she gets out of or into bed. The nurse provides the touch cue by moving into contact with Mrs Polanszky – and into her personal space.

TO MOVE ALONG THE EDGE OF THE BED

A nurse sits down at Mrs Polanszky's side and asks her to 'Move along, please'; at the same time she gives her a gentle nudge with her hip. Mrs Polanszky moves away from her. The nurse repeats the nudge several times so that Mrs Polanszky gradually moves along the edge, from one end of the bed to the other.

Advantages of this strategy   The movement promoted by the strategy is a very safe one, because the person remains in the sitting position throughout. It is also an excellent source of exercise when carried out regularly (see exercise suggestions in Chapter 10).

Disadvantages   It is possible that a very small person might feel intimidated by a large assistant who uses this strategy. So an alternative strategy is sometimes required. In this case, the assistant can use the palms of both hands to give a 'move-along' touch cue to the person's nearer hip. The hand pressure needs to be positive and may need to be kept up for a couple of seconds in order to persuade the person to move along the edge of the bed.

Touch while giving physical support

The importance of giving help in a safe and effective way was dealt with in Chapter 5. In it you were introduced to the palm-to-palm thumb hold; to the importance of getting close to someone when you help them; and to the advantages of providing a firm pillar of support to help someone to rise from the sitting position.

When you give someone physical support you need to use the whole length of your arms, as well as your body. Workers who move and handle heavy loads are advised to hold the load close to their bodies; the same guidance applies to you. You must get into close contact with the individual in a matter-of-fact professional way, so that you avoid the possibility of its being interpreted as a sexual approach. Physiotherapists often need to get onto the treatment couch alongside the person in order to carry out their work. They have to be particularly careful that their actions are not misunderstood.

USING TOUCH FOR EXTRA REASSURANCE

Mr Cash needs help to walk. The nurse supports him closely so that she can walk 'in unison' with him. She uses the palm-to-palm thumb hold with one hand and holds onto the handling belt he is wearing with her other hand. On this side, her hand and arm and the side of her body and hip are in contact with his body. The support she gives is comfortable and kindly; it reassures him and makes him feel safe. Mr Cash suddenly says that he is afraid of falling – he seems to have forgotten that the nurse is supporting him. She immediately adds a comforting squeeze to the hand that she is supporting. Mr Cash is reassured by this extra touch and he continues his walk.

Touch for silent communication

Most touch cues that you give add meaning to your spoken requests. They give a silent message about the direction of the movement required. Touch can convey silent messages of another kind: those that show praise, sympathy, reassurance and caring. It is not easy to describe these silent messages in words, but you can congratulate or praise someone with a pat on the back or a quick hug; sympathy with a hand quietly placed on a shoulder; reassurance with a comforting squeeze of the hand or arm; and caring by holding a hand.

Using touch to relax/calm

It is possible for normally calm people to become agitated; sometimes you know the cause, sometimes you do not. When people are agitated they are less likely to co-operate with you; they may refuse to move or to carry out the task that you ask them to do. So it is useful to be able to calm them with a soothing hand massage. You need relaxed hands for this.

GIVING A HAND MASSAGE

Mrs Polanszky sometimes becomes distressed when she does not understand what the nurses want her to do. Anna, the Polish nurse, can comfort her with a short hand massage. She seats herself facing Mrs Polanszky but to one side so that she can see her face and reach her nearer hand comfortably. She takes Mrs Polanszky's hand, palm down, in one of her own, and supports it on the chair arm (or on her knees if the chair arm is not comfortable). She then rests her other hand on top and starts to make tiny stroking movements slowly over the back of Mrs Polanszky's hand. She strokes from the wrist towards the fingers, then lifts her hand and returns rhythmically to the wrist area. She keeps her hand relaxed so that it follows the shape of Mrs Polanszky's hand.

Anna carries on with the gentle stroking until Mrs Polanszky becomes calmer. She continues for a few more minutes, gradually coming to a stop by lengthening the strokes and making them less frequent. She then sits quietly at Mrs Polanszky's side before moving away – gently encouraging her to rest awhile. She returns later to help her to carry out the movement or task originally requested.

Using touch to release a grip

The use of the palm-to-palm thumb hold, described on page 54, prevents people from gripping the arms of their chair when they are asked to stand up. This method of supporting hands is very effective indeed, but how do you persuade a frightened person to let go of the chair arms?

SETTING OUT TO RELEASE THE GRIP

You can start by asking, 'Give me your hand, please?' or 'Put your hand in [or on] mine?', and providing a cue by offering him your hand, palm up. If repeated requests do not succeed, you need to gently lift the hand off. Pulling his hand off just makes matters worse and you could hurt it by squeezing, especially if he has painful joints. You can, however, make use of a reflex to release the grip instead.

RELEASING THE GRIPPING HAND

Position yourself at the person's side as if you were about to give a touch cue (see Chapter 3) and place your 'inner' hand (the one that you usually use for supporting him at waist or hip level) at the back of his upper arm, just below the shoulder. Slide this hand, smoothly, down the back of his arm to the wrist. Your hand slides over any clothing and finishes up between the chair arm and his lower arm. Cradle his wrist in your hand. Then, using your other hand, stroke the back of his hand towards the fingers, a couple of times, briskly but lightly. As soon as you have done this, you should be able to lift his hand gently off the chair arm with your 'cradling' hand. You can now take up the palm-to-palm thumb hold by placing your 'outer' hand, palm up, under his hand.

Taking up the hold when the person is standing You can use the same method of taking up the palm-to-palm thumb hold when someone is standing up. In this case there is no gripping to overcome. You merely place your inner hand under the person's elbow and slide it down to the wrist so that you support his arm while you take up the palm-to-palm thumb hold with your outer hand.

Conclusion

Touch can convey many different messages. Some people use it more than others, but it should always be done for a purpose. Sometimes touching becomes a meaningless personal habit that can be very irritating to the person receiving it. Other people find touching difficult; they have to overcome their reluctance and learn how to use it with confidence.

Everyone who works with people with dementia needs to be aware of what they say and how they say it. They should also be aware of what they are doing with their hands while they are speaking.

KEY POINTS

- Use touch thoughtfully.
- Relax your hands for greatest effect.
- Encourage movement with touch cues.
- Use touch to convey your feelings.

TRAINING EXERCISES

Working with a colleague:

1 Practise the brief relaxation routine in Appendix 1.

2 Practise giving a hand massage to your colleague (see p 84).

3 Practise using touch to release a grip and taking up the palm-to-palm hold (see p 85).

Reference

Mitchell, Laura (1977) *Simple Relaxation.* John Murray, London

9 Seeking Professional Help

This chapter stresses the need for a team approach. It looks briefly at ways in which staff are organised in order to promote effective communication and good practice. It explains how the services of an occupational therapist or a physiotherapist are normally obtained, the services they provide and some examples of the problems that they can deal with.

The team

Dementia care needs a team approach with everyone working towards the same goals. Many services are now organised from teams in the community. These can be based in either a general medical practice or a community mental health centre. Assessment, guidance and support are provided by a team of professional workers who are skilled in different aspects of dementia care.

Key-workers

A key-worker is usually responsible for co-ordinating the person's package of care in the community. This worker keeps in touch with her clients even if they are admitted to hospital for assessment or treatment.

Named nurses

Most people who are being cared for in a hospital, nursing or residential home have a named nurse. In a hospital or nursing home, this person has a nursing qualification. The named nurse stays in close touch with the key-workers in the team and is likely to be responsible for several nurses or care staff who look after the same group of people. This means that, when the named nurse is not on duty, there is always someone available who is familiar with their care. In a small nursing home, when the named nurse is not on duty, queries from visiting professional staff or relatives are likely to be dealt with by the matron or the officer in charge. These arrangements help to promote good standards of nursing practice. Make sure that communication is as good as possible; it is a vital part of the caring process.

Gaining access to help and advice

If someone you are caring for is having difficulties with mobility, you are likely to be looking for help from an occupational therapist or a physiotherapist. In some situations, this specialised professional support is routinely provided when it is needed. This is likely to occur in a hospital's mental health assessment unit or in the day hospital attached to it.

Nursing and residential homes

Some nursing and residential homes are able to obtain help from community therapists, whereas others employ their own. People in private nursing care often have to pay extra for these services and for the hire of any walking equipment that is needed.

Carers

Carers can reach the occupational therapy or physiotherapy services through their general practitioner. However, these community-based services are always very much in demand and there may be a waiting list.

Occupational therapist or physiotherapist?

There is often some overlap between the roles of occupational therapists and physiotherapists who work with people with dementia.

Occupational therapist

An occupational therapist is more likely to use her skills with assessing and planning programmes for people who have difficulty in feeding, dressing, bathing, toileting, cooking, cleaning and shopping, and with the mobility that is needed for these tasks.

Physiotherapist

A physiotherapist is more likely to be assessing and interpreting the problems of people who find the basic activities of daily living difficult – for example, movement from a bed or chair, walking and transfers.

Advice on footwear, seating, walking aids, wheelchairs, hoists and on moving and handling problems for people with dementia may be given by either therapist, or in the case of footwear by a chiropodist. These topics are dealt with more fully later in this chapter.

Note The organisation of these services can vary greatly from one area to another.

Working with the therapist

A detailed assessment is always carried out by the therapist before she gives you any advice or supplies you with any equipment that you might request. She needs to see for herself what the person's problems are, and to find out why he has them. She is then in a position to discuss the matter with you and to suggest what might be done to ease them.

Providing information

In order to carry out the assessment, the therapist needs medical details about the person as well as any useful information from you or from his relatives. The therapist must know what drugs he is taking, because some of these may be affecting his mobility or his behaviour. She may prefer to carry out the assessment quietly on her own, but be prepared to stay with her and help if necessary. If you are present, let the therapist do the talking, so that the person is not confused by two different voices. And stay silent if he seems to be willing to move for the therapist although he normally refuses to do so for you. Save your comments for later when you are out of his sight and earshot.

Where should the assessment take place?

The best place for the assessment is in the person's own home, in familiar surroundings with familiar objects around him. But, if he is living and being cared for in a residential or nursing home, that is where it should take place. His bedroom is probably the best spot: it is private and quiet. Prepare him by telling him to expect a special visitor, even if you are fairly certain that he will forget about it. You can then remind him from time to time – he may refuse to co-operate if he is not well prepared.

How long does it take?

The assessment process is likely to take more than one visit – getting to know the individual takes time, and he may not be at his best on the first occasion. The therapist also has to make allowances for any variations in his ability to carry out tasks at different times of the day.

Discussing the results of the assessment

The therapist needs to discuss her findings with you. The assessment shows what the person can and cannot do. In some cases, it is obvious that he is able to do the movement but does not carry it out for some reason. The therapist then has to decide what is making him behave in this way – you can help by giving her your opinion. Does he understand what he is being asked to do? Is he afraid to move? Is he in pain? These problems were looked at in detail in earlier chapters and suggestions were made about how to deal with them.

Agreeing goals

When the therapist decides what action is needed, she is able to suggest some goals. She will negotiate with you about them; you need to work together to achieve most of the goals. For example, she finds that the person cannot stand up straight because the muscles around his hips are tight. The goal will be to make standing upright possible again. She suggests that this can be achieved if he is given a stretch on the bed once a day. Together, you might agree that the best time for lying flat on the bed is soon after lunch – and this is added to his care plan.

WRITTEN REPORTS

You should expect to receive a written report from the therapist within a reasonable length of time, but it is a wise move to get her to jot down the main points of her advice immediately – it is easy to forget what has been said when you are busy.

When should you seek help?

You need to seek help from a physiotherapist if someone's mobility is severely limited; if his ability to walk suddenly deteriorates for no obvious reason; if he has difficulty in regaining mobility following a period in bed or after fractures and strokes; when he has problems with walking, balance and posture; and for stretching out and preventing any shortened muscles (see 'contractures' in the Glossary).

Your involvement

While someone is receiving therapy, you are likely to be asked to give him the opportunity to practise different tasks during the course of the day. The physiotherapist will advise you what you can do to help achieve the goals and ask you to supervise the use of any equipment supplied.

PRACTISING A PARTICULAR ACTIVITY

Mr Cash has become rather anxious about approaching and sitting down on a chair. The physiotherapist is asked to assess him. She finds that he is better at approaching the chair when it is on his left than when it is on his right – his vision is not good but he can see the chair more clearly when it is on his left side. She asks his nurse to help him on his right side, so that the chair will be on his left when he approaches it. From this position he can see the chair and reach for the arm-rest more easily. He soon becomes less anxious.

USING WALKING EQUIPMENT

Mrs Polanszky's arthritic knees are making walking difficult for her – she leans heavily on the nurses. Anna, her named nurse, feels that a walking aid of some sort might be helpful. The physiotherapist assesses Mrs Polanszky and agrees with her – they decide to try a walking aid with wheels. Anna alters Mrs Polanszky's care plan so that other members of staff know about the trial use of the equipment. The walking aid is a success, so it is issued for permanent use by Mrs Polanskzy, with supervision.

FITTING A SPLINT

Miss Kenny is having difficulty in holding her spoon at meal times – it slips out of her hand. The nurses have tried using one with a padded handle, but this does not help her. The doctor diagnoses a 'dropped wrist' and asks an occupational therapist for her help; the nerve serving the muscles has been damaged. Miss Kenny tends to doze in her chair and sometimes leans heavily against her arm, which she traps between her body and the wooden arm-rest. The visiting occupational therapist makes a little splint to support the wrist in a good position while the nerve recovers. She fits it and Miss Kenny is immediately able to hold her spoon once more. The splint has to be carefully applied and kept in place with a series of soft straps. It has to be removed at night and refitted each morning, so the occupational therapist shows the nursing staff how to do this. She also stresses the need to check that the skin does not become sore. She explains that the splint will be worn less and less once the nerve starts to recover.

Obtaining advice

Therapists are able to give you advice on other problems, such as footwear, seating, the use of hoists, and moving and handling. They are also able to provide, or to advise you how to obtain, special footwear and seating, and equipment such as walking aids and wheelchairs. The guidance and comments given below, on footwear, seating and walking aids, should help you to make some decisions on your own.

Footwear

Shoes that are comfortable and give plenty of support to your feet are a pleasure to wear. You probably have a favourite pair of 'lace-ups', for work or for walking, which keep your feet firmly in place on the soles. Older people also benefit from wearing well-fitting shoes, even if they only walk short distances indoors. Slippers make walking much more difficult for them.

SLIPPERS AND 'TRAINERS'

Many people like to wear slippers during the day instead of shoes. These do not support their feet and allow them to slip off the soles onto the uppers. It is not unusual to see an older person struggling to walk with his slippers half off, making walking unnecessarily difficult and danger-ous. Bootee slippers cannot slide off in the same way, but their soles are very soft. These tend to stick to the floor and do not allow the wearer to slide his foot forwards when it comes into contact with the floor. We all need to do this sometimes when we stub the toe of our footwear. Unfor-tunately, the soles of 'trainers' behave in a similar way. So this and the flatness of their soles also make trainers unsuitable for older people who walk with difficulty.

SANDALS

To condemn all sandals as unsuitable is not wise, because styles can vary so much. 'Strappy' sandals and 'sling-backs' (see Glossary) are not suit-able, nor are those with spongy soles. The ones that are more like shoes may be acceptable if they support the feet well, are not too flat and have leather or firm composition soles.

SHOES

A securely fastened, well-fitting shoe helps you to balance by supporting your foot on the sole. Most people prefer to wear shoes with a small heel rather than completely flat ones. Older people who have mobility prob-lems certainly need shoes with a broad heel that gives them a good base to walk on. Shoes also provide some protection from accidental knocks and prevent damage to their feet, if they happen to step on some small object on the floor. For these reasons, walking with bare feet can be hazardous.

Men's shoes   The traditional style of men's shoes, lace-ups or slip-ons, with nice broad heels, are usually suitable for people whose feet are in good condition. Relatives or friends are often able to bring a selection of the person's own shoes for you to look at. There may be a suitable pair in good condition among them; the uppers must not be misshapen and the soles and heels not worn down unevenly. Ask the individual which pair he prefers to wear, or ask his relatives.

Women's shoes   Finding suitable shoes for women is usually more difficult. Many of the shoes in their wardrobe are fashionable and do not offer the necessary support. Court shoes and strappy sandals are not suitable. You may, however, be lucky enough to find a couple of pairs of 'flat' ones with medium-height broad heels that fit and are in good condition. If this is the case, allow the woman to choose which ones she prefers.

Miss Kenny provides us with an example of how the lack of a heel can affect women who have always worn high-heeled shoes. Before she was admitted to the local authority home, Miss Kenny was walking unaided. When she was admitted, however, the nurses found that she walked unsteadily and needed their help to move about. She was wearing the flat-soled slippers sent in by her friend.

The physiotherapist assessed her and found that the muscles at the back of the calves of her legs were tight. This tightness was stopping her from putting her heels to the floor and making her walk on her toes. Miss Kenny's friend was asked to bring in some of her shoes, and a pair with a broad high-ish heel was chosen. The heels made it possible for Miss Kenny to put both feet flat on the floor and to walk steadily without support. She just needed someone beside her to help her find her way about. The friend confirmed that Miss Kenny had worn smart, high-heeled shoes all her adult life.

Buying new shoes   You will be anxious to spare relatives the expense of buying new shoes, if at all possible. However, if you or the therapist are not satisfied that 'old friends' are suitable, new ones will be needed. A leather upper is better than a man-made one, because it moulds much better to the shape of the foot; it also allows the feet to 'breathe' and reduces sweating. Style and colour also matter to women, so seek their opinion as well as that of the relatives who are paying for the new footwear. You may need to persuade the relatives of the benefits of shoes – of the improved safety and ease of walking.

Shoes for problem feet can be expensive but are now available in a choice of attractive styles and colours. Modifications to shoes (see Glossary) and the supply of surgical footwear may be arranged free of charge through the National Health Service.

GENERAL GUIDANCE ON FOOTWEAR

- Check the condition of the person's feet as well as of their shoes. Use your common sense for this; if you have any doubts, seek the advice of a chiropodist.
- Never allow someone to wear shoes without socks or tights.
- Remember that some people may not have worn shoes for some time. So, whether the shoes are old or new, carry out a slow *wearing-in* period: allow them to wear the shoes for an hour to start with and then gradually increase the time.
- Do not hesitate to seek help; a more experienced colleague may be able to guide you, but, if you are in doubt, contact your therapist or a chiropodist before you act.

Seating

The type of chair a person sits in can affect his ability to rise. An unsuitable chair, such as a very low one or a big heavy armchair with a deep soft seat, can turn an active person into a prisoner. The wide padded arms of some chairs also make it difficult for you to give help effectively: you cannot get close enough to him and that puts your back at risk of injury. A well-chosen chair may make it possible for him to rise without help, or to be helped from it much more easily (see Chapter 7 – Mr Cash). So when seating is being chosen, the needs of both the people themselves and the people who care for them have to be considered. Hospital units, day hospitals, and nursing and residential homes should be able to offer a selection of different sizes and styles to cater for different needs.

COLOUR OF THE UPHOLSTERY

It is much easier for people with dementia and those who care for them to pick out chairs of a particular seat height if they are upholstered in the same colour. So a lounge with chairs of two or three different heights could contain chairs in two or three different colours, according to their height. It is worth bearing in mind that, for people with poor eyesight, chairs upholstered in exactly the same colour as the carpet seem to disappear into it.

SEATING PROBLEMS

You should seek the advice of an occupational therapist or physiotherapist about seating problems. The Disabled Living Foundation, or the local equivalent (often called 'disabled living centres'), also provides information about seating. There are, however, a few general checks that you can make yourself on an individual's easy chair.

1 Start with the chair empty, on a non-slip surface or wedged against the wall, and kneel on the seat. Can you feel the framework underneath your knees? If you can, the chair will not be comfortable to sit on.
2 Now seat the person in the chair and check him from the side and the front. Does he look comfortable and well supported?
3 When his feet are flat on the floor, does the seat support the full length of his thighs, without causing any undue pressure at the back of his knees?
4 Can he rest *back* against the back-rest? It should slope backwards a little.
5 Is his back fully supported by the back-rest, especially in the low back (lumbar) region? Is his head also supported?
6 Does the seat slope a few degrees towards the chair back? Is this enough to prevent him from sliding out of it? (A slope of 6–8 degrees is normal.)
7 Do the arm-rests support his lower arms comfortably without pushing his shoulders up?
8 Is there enough space under the front of the chair seat to allow him to pull his feet back when he prepares to rise?

Walking aids

People who have difficulty walking are most likely to be issued with an aid with or without wheels.

WALKING FRAMES

A walking frame has to be used in a co-ordinated way: it must be lifted forward each time and then stepped into, in a lift–step–step pattern. Someone using a walking frame has to balance without support while he lifts it forward. For this reason many people find a frame with wheels easier to manage.

FRAMES WITH WHEELS

These are pushed along the floor or the ground, but they can also be lifted up and used like a walking frame if the need arises. People using a frame with wheels usually push it ahead until their elbows are straight and then they step into it. You can encourage or help them to use a push–step–step pattern to move over level surfaces, and to lift it over any prominent threshold strips or other changes in floor level.

There are several different types of wheeled frames: the ones that have a *braking system* built into their wheels are safest – those with *hand-controlled brakes* are usually too complicated for people with dementia. Brakes are essential to stop wheeled equipment from running away. If the equipment is used correctly, the brakes in the wheels work automatically. They operate when the person using the frame presses down on it.

Warning The braking system built into the wheels cannot operate if the aid is pushed too far forward.

WALKING STICKS

These are not often useful in units where there are other people. Sticks make good weapons; they get lost; they are difficult to 'park'; and they are a danger to others when they fall or are placed on the floor. This is a Health and Safety issue, so if someone insists on having a stick, you must assess the risk and then come to a decision – involve the person concerned.

People who are being cared for at home might well use one successfully there. In that case, only one stick should be provided – the use of two sticks requires a high degree of co-ordination. Walking sticks are available in two styles: those with a hooked top and those with only a knob. Choose the one with the hook so that there is some chance of hanging it over the arm of a chair where it will be less of a hazard. You will have to remind the person to use it, because he is likely to forget it.

Warning Rubber ferrules on any piece of walking equipment can wear down and make it unsafe to use. Check them regularly and replace them if they have worn down and become smooth.

Height of equipment

The therapist who assesses the person also supplies or makes arrangements for the supply of the walking aid. She decides which type of aid is required and fixes its height, so you must never use equipment issued to one person for someone else. Attach a label to each item so that this does not happen.

CHECKING THE HEIGHT

Much of this equipment is height adjustable. Some types have a screw adjuster which can work loose or be turned by the person using it; it is important that you check these from time to time. Although the therapist is responsible for deciding the height of the aid, you should be able to make an emergency adjustment if the need arises. You need a tape-measure before you start.

1 Ask the person to stand and hold onto something solid, such as the dining table.
2 Get him to take one hand off the support and place his arm at his side.
3 Measure from his wrist, just below the prominent bone on the little finger side of the back of his hand, down to the floor.
4 Re-seat him.
5 Compare this measurement with the height of the walking aid at the hand grips.
6 Adjust the height and tighten the screws firmly.
7 Report the problem to the therapist.

In addition to checking the equipment from time to time, you also need to make arrangements for it to be kept clean.

KEY POINTS

- Recognise the importance of a team approach.
- Recognise the value of working together towards common goals.
- Recognise the benefits of suitable footwear and seating.

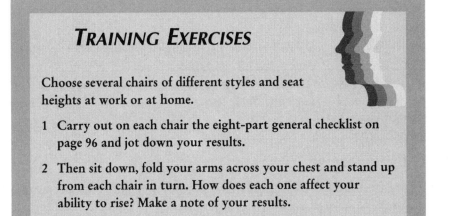

TRAINING EXERCISES

Choose several chairs of different styles and seat heights at work or at home.

1 Carry out on each chair the eight-part general checklist on page 96 and jot down your results.

2 Then sit down, fold your arms across your chest and stand up from each chair in turn. How does each one affect your ability to rise? Make a note of your results.

10 Exercise

Exercise can be used to achieve many different aims. This chapter looks at some of them and suggests how levels of exercise can be varied to suit the needs of individual people. It also looks at the causes of falls and considers the problems of restlessness and wandering.

Daily exercise

Exercise can benefit older people in many different ways. It can increase their fitness, strengthen muscles, loosen joints and stimulate or relax their mind and body. It can relieve boredom and restlessness, act as a release from frustration and stress, and provide a source of enjoyment and fun.

What sort of exercise is suitable for people with dementia?

All the basic daily activities (rising to standing, walking, sitting down, transferring, moving on, off and across a bed, using steps and stairs) that have been described in this book can provide a source of exercise. They form part of daily life, so they are familiar and mean something to people with dementia – which is very important. They make it possible for you to promote mobility and improve balance with exercise that is part of the daily routine. Previous chapters in this book showed you how to talk to the people you are caring for and how, with a variety of different strategies and approaches, to motivate them to move.

The effects of inactivity

Older people are usually less active than they were when they were younger. Many of them spend more time sitting down and are reluctant to take exercise. The results of this inactivity are weaker muscles and stiffer joints. Weak muscles lead to unsteadiness and falls, with the risk of fractures. This risk becomes even greater when bones have become thin because of osteoporosis.

Falls

Many people with dementia fall. Sometimes it is obvious why they have fallen, but on many occasions the reason is not so clear. Whatever the cause, the effect of a fall can be far-reaching. Even if there are no physical injuries, the shock and distress are great and confidence is shattered. As a result, the person is very much at risk of 'going off their feet' unless action is taken to prevent this from happening.

When there are injuries, such as a fracture, surgery and a long period of rehabilitation are needed if the person is to have any chance of regaining some mobility – this is an expensive business. Sadly, some people do not survive the surgery and others may not receive – or even be offered – the physiotherapy they need.

HIP PADS

It is extremely difficult to prevent falls in people with dementia who are prone to falling but who are able to move about on their own. If they do fall, it is their hips that are likely to be fractured. It is possible, however, to protect their hips with padding – this has been done successfully in Sweden and has started in the UK. So, in the near future, many more older people may be fitted with hip pads; the shock of the fall will remain, but a costly fracture may be prevented.

You can see that the prevention of falls is a very important matter. A great deal of research has recently taken place into this subject, and it is now clear that there are many causes, or combinations of causes. We will look at the more obvious causes first, and then at the ones that researchers tell us about.

Obvious causes

These are the ones that most people think about when the causes of falls are mentioned: the edge of a carpet, the wet patch or food spilt on a hard floor, the loose sole of a shoe or slipper, poor lighting hiding a step and other similar hazards. Then there is poor eyesight and the wearing of unsuitable glasses. You can make sure that action is taken to remove any such hazards and that only appropriate glasses are worn.

Main causes

These include the side-effects of medication, poor general health, the effects of dementia and impaired balance and mobility. You can contribute to the prevention of falls in several ways, as outlined below.

SIDE-EFFECTS OF MEDICATION

Ask the doctor to review the person's medication, especially if you think that it is making him giddy or unsteady. It may be possible for the doctor to give him a similar drug that has fewer side-effects.

EFFECTS OF DEMENTIA

Make sure that you reduce to a minimum any features in the person's surroundings that might be misinterpreted or cause 'stepping' (see Chapter 6).

IMPAIRED BALANCE AND MOBILITY

Balance and mobility are affected if muscles are weak. So it is important for people with dementia to regain, maintain or improve their muscle power. You can help them by gradually stepping up their exercise, not only to reduce the risk of falls and fractures but also for all the many benefits of remaining mobile (see Chapter 1).

Forward planning

Falls usually occur when the person is walking, so before setting out make a few quick checks and preparations:

- Make sure that the floor is clear of anything that he might trip over, such as a fallen walking stick, the strap of a handbag, a discarded slipper, a child's toy, a trailing electric cable.
- Place a chair at the half-way mark of a short walk, as a possible resting place. If the distance is longer or the person cannot see the 'goal

chair' because it is in another room, place other chairs along the route so that he can always see and walk towards one. It is better for him to complete the walk safely with rests on the way than to risk a fall. As an alternative, ask a colleague to follow you with a wheelchair.

- Open any doors that you have to pass through or arrange for someone to hold them open for you, and make sure that the way is well lit.
- Check that the person is wearing his hearing aid and his glasses, if he needs them, and that the hearing aid is working properly – being able to communicate with him is essential.
- Make sure that his shoes are fastened securely and that he is wearing a belt or braces to hold up his trousers.

WHAT YOU SHOULD DO IF THE PERSON YOU ARE HELPING STARTS TO FALL

If you are helping someone to move and he tells you that he is going to fall, say very firmly: 'Stand up . . . Stay standing', as described on page 18. If he does not do this immediately, you must *lower* him to the ground, as described below. *Do not try to hold him up* – you could seriously injure your back.

If, on the other hand, his legs begin to collapse and he starts to fall, you must lower him to the floor immediately. *You must not attempt to hold him up or to 'catch' him.*

You should receive training in how to lower someone to the floor and then practise the sequence regularly. The moves are:

- Release yourself from the hold you are using.
- Move quickly behind him.
- Open your hands, palms upwards, and take one step backwards.
- Allow the falling person to slide down your body onto the floor, guiding him with your open hands. Do not try to soften his descent by hanging onto him or his clothing.
- If the person is uninjured and able to get up by himself, he can do so from here (see the guidance given below). Otherwise, lie him down, make him comfortable and *use a hoist to lift him* off the floor.

HOW TO 'TALK' A PERSON UP FROM THE FLOOR

If you know that the person can get up off the floor by himself, first of all ask him calmly to 'Stand up, please' – he may do so automatically, without thinking about it. Do not rush him, give him plenty of time. If he does not get up, you need to be able to tell him what to do, but do *not* be tempted to give him any help.

• Place a stout chair close to him.
• Tell him to turn onto his side towards the chair – this gives him a visual cue. He should now be sitting on one side and turned towards the chair.
• Get him to lean on the seat of the chair with one arm – pat the seat to show him where – and to pull himself up onto his knees.
• Tell him to put his other hand on the seat or the arm of the chair – pat it if necessary – and urge him to 'Stand up' (this is probably more effective than 'Get up', but try either) – and to pull himself up onto his feet.
• Now he can either turn to sit down on this chair or you can avoid the difficult turn involved by placing a chair behind him.

How much exercise is needed?

People with dementia have different strengths and weaknesses, so their needs are going to vary. Although the planned level of exercise will be different for each individual, most of them benefit from a short daily session of exercises in a group – either music and movement or activities with small pieces of interesting equipment (see Chapter 7).

Relatively mobile people

People who are able to carry out most of the basic daily activities with or without help are likely to need further exercise to maintain their muscle strength. An excellent way of achieving this is to gradually increase the distance they are able to walk; walking outside is particularly beneficial because walking balance is more difficult on the uneven surface. In the following example an increase in the number of times that the person walks is used to provide extra exercise.

INCREASING THE AMOUNT OF EXERCISE

Mr Patel had, you remember, started to grab at door frames when passing through doorways (see Chapter 5). Mrs Patel is using a strategy to deal with this problem. But she is still worried that her husband might not continue to be able to manage the stairs; she does not want to have the bed downstairs in their small lounge. She discusses her worries with Mark, their community psychiatric nurse. They take a careful look at Mr Patel's day and decide to increase his activity.

Stepping up the frequency of walking

Mrs Patel always serves drinks and meals on a little table beside her husband's chair, so that he does not have to move out of it. They agree that this pattern needs to be changed – Mr Patel ought to walk to the dining table instead. She starts by taking him to the table for the main meals of the day, and then, over a period of time, adds all coffee, tea and other drink breaks as well. This provides him with much more exercise.

Within eight weeks Mr Patel is walking with more confidence. His present level of activity is maintaining his strength and he continues to manage the stairs.

Less mobile people

People who are less mobile have difficulty in walking and in carrying out some of the other basic daily activities. In this case, you need to set down what you think they are doing and then check that they are in fact doing it – you will need to use a checklist. This gives you a baseline of activity, which you are then able to increase very gradually. You can use any of the basic daily activities to increase their exercise. The example below shows you how you might achieve this.

INCREASING THE USE OF TRANSFERS

If someone is finding it difficult to walk more than a few steps, it is better to provide extra exercise by increasing the use of transfers than to expect him to walk more often or to increase the distance he walks. For example, at mealtimes, aim to get him to transfer from his easy chair into a wheelchair and to transfer from the wheelchair to a dining chair when you reach the table. This simple strategy starts to give him many more opportunities for movement and exercise.

SUGGESTED EXERCISES

Make sure that *everyone* who is less mobile maintains their ability to do the following.

- Move along the edge of the bed, in the sitting position, until the end is reached, on getting up or going to bed (see p 82). This provides a source of safe exercise and strengthens the muscles needed for standing up from a chair.
- Carry out transfers regularly. This makes moving from seat to seat possible without the aid of a hoist.
- Sit on a padded stool or low table for about 15 minutes daily. This helps to maintain the ability to sit upright, and to prevent backward leaning. Encourage him to turn his head or his body occasionally, for example to look at a book. **Warning:** someone must stay with the person throughout.
- Balance in the standing position for one minute, without support if possible. Place the back of a chair or a walking aid in the space in front of him to give added security and confidence. Encourage him to turn his head or body to look around him while he is balancing.

Relatively immobile people

You are, of course, aiming to maintain the best levels of mobility in everyone. However, in spite of your best efforts and that of the physiotherapist, some people do become increasingly less mobile. In these cases, you aim to maintain some mobility and to prevent the unnecessary onset of any of the problems that accompany immobility by:

- Maintaining the ability to stand to a support for one minute – this helps nursing care, gives the person the opportunity to put some weight on his feet, gives some pressure relief and helps to prevent him becoming permanently 'chair-shaped'.
- Allowing the person to lie flat on the bed for 20–30 minutes in the

middle of the day – this can give him a good stretch and helps prevent the development of contractures (see Glossary). It also gives his neck muscles a well-deserved rest. The head is very heavy and the neck muscles may not be strong enough to hold it up all day; the back-rest of a chair gives only partial support to the head.

Exercise to reduce boredom

You need to provide enough stimulation for people during the day. A lack of it may result in some of them becoming bored and restless. The ones who wander about may be doing so to relieve their boredom; your assessment will show you whether this is likely. In this case, it is worth while introducing some structured activities into their day, to see if the wandering lessens. Try to persuade them to join in with the daily session of group exercises and to occupy them with other activities during the day (see Chapter 7).

Some hospitals are fortunate enough to have a 'sensory room' with comfortable seating, where people can enjoy watching moving lights and listening to sounds. This provides a different and interesting source of stimulation.

Managing restlessness or wandering

It is essential to assess each person to find the causes of the restless or wandering behaviour. Only then is it possible to seek solutions for it – with skilful management you should be able to reduce the severity of the behaviour. Restraint is not acceptable; it may cause a violent response or result in a loss of mobility.

Boredom is only one of the causes; others can be physical, environmental or emotional. There are often several combined causes.

PHYSICAL CAUSES

Some people may be in pain or suffering some other discomfort, such as constipation, and, because they cannot explain this in words, they try to get away from it. Treatment of such problems should result in more relaxed people.

It is also possible for medication to be the cause of the restlessness; the doctor may be able to change it or reduce the dosage.

People who are restless when seated may need a more suitable chair. Ask the occupational therapist or physiotherapist to assess them for you. A special chair may solve the problem.

ENVIRONMENTAL CAUSES

There may be too much stimulation in a person's immediate surroundings. He may be trying to escape from an area that is too hot or too noisy, or from someone who is upsetting him. You can probably arrange for him to spend some of his time in a quieter area.

The surroundings may be unfamiliar and confusing to him. In this case, he may respond to your efforts to help him become more familiar with them. He will also need plenty of frequent reassurance.

EMOTIONAL CAUSES

He may feel lost and agitated, and be looking for someone or something familiar; he needs reassurance and understanding. Try to build up a trusting relationship with him by using touch, in the form of a hand massage, to calm and reassure him (see Chapter 8).

He may be anxious, and goes for a walk – many people do this when they want to sort out their worries. If you spend time with him and watch his body language for cues, you may be able to find out what is worrying him.

Conclusion

The pieces of the jigsaw are now laid out for you to see. They are all different but they fit together to make a complete picture. They can, in fact, be arranged in different ways so that you can create many different pictures with them. Sometimes you will need all the pieces, and on other occasions only a few. If one piece does not fit, look for a similar one and try that instead. Does it fit better? The more familiar you become with the jigsaw, the easier it becomes to fit the pieces together.

This mobility jigsaw forms a small part of the overall concept of good practice in dementia care.

KEY POINTS

- Muscle weakness causes falls.
- Exercise strengthens muscles.
- Make exercise part of the daily routine.
- Provide opportunities for extra exercise.
- Give mobility a high priority.
- Seek the causes of restlessness and wandering.

11 Points to Remember

- Many strategies and approaches have been suggested in the preceding chapters. Each one has been used successfully with people with dementia.
- There are no guarantees of success, but the strategies and approaches described in this book are likely to lessen the difficulties of the people you are caring for and ease the problems facing you.
- Each person is an individual with his own set of difficulties and needs, so you are unlikely to be using the same strategies with everyone.
- Watch people's reactions carefully, so that you can change your approach if necessary.
- Remember that individuals may react differently to different people.
- The environment makes a big impact on people with dementia; it can increase or decrease their willingness or ability to move about in it.
- Bear in mind that the abilities and reactions of people with dementia may vary from hour to hour as well as from day to day.

You will find lists of strategies in Appendix 2. For ease of use they are presented under each everyday activity.

APPENDIX 1 BRIEF RELAXATION ROUTINE

Position

Standing up with your arms at your sides

Method

Carry out the movements in the same order each time you use the routine.

- Carry out the movement.
- Stop doing the movement.
- Pause, then start the next movement.

Movements

1 *Pull your shoulders down towards the floor* You should feel them 'bounce' back a little when you stop doing the movement.
2 *Stretch out your fingers, thumbs and wrists* After you stop, your fingers will become very slightly curved.
3 *Start a yawn, or 'pull your jaw down'* When you stop, your top and bottom teeth should stay slightly apart.
4 *Tell yourself to smooth out the worry lines across your forehead and the 'frown' lines at the bridge of your nose* This is not a movement like the others. When you stop, your forehead should feel smooth and the bridge of your nose 'wide'.

Result

Your shoulders, hands and face should now feel more relaxed. Repeat the routine once more if you feel that your face in particular needs a little more attention. The whole routine should take you only a few seconds to complete each time.

APPENDIX 2 LISTS OF STRATEGIES

Communication strategies

Initial approach

- Approach the person slowly from the front.
- Respect his personal space.
- Address him by name and make eye contact.
- Keep your hand and body movements smooth and unhurried.
- Speak clearly, in a manner acceptable to an adult.
- Make use of facial expression.
- Be courteous.

Verbal strategies

- Give the person plenty of time.
- Use short sentences.
- Limit requests to one at a time.
- Use repetition, and change wording if necessary.
- Experiment with words and expressions.
- Avoid inviting a refusal.
- Word requests in a positive way.
- Give step-by-step instructions if helpful.
- Word requests for an automatic response.
- Use tone of voice to suggest the ease of the task.
- Listen to what you say and watch the person's reactions.

Note When there are two assistants, only one should speak.

From Appendix 2 of *Promoting Mobility for People with Dementia:
A problem-solving approach* by Rosemary Oddy.
You may copy this page.

Sitting to standing

- Plan to succeed.
- Be positive and understanding.
- Think while you give help.

General points

- Seating.
- Footwear and clothes.
- Hearing aids and dentures.
- Spectacles.

Suggested strategies

- Place a chair in the space in front of the person.
- Ask him to rise, firmly and politely or lightly and casually to suggest the ease of the task.
- Use a gesture to indicate the need to rise.
- Use a stationary touch cue or sweep your hand up the person's back.
- Place his hands on the chair arms as a cue to the movement.
- Use a goal-based cue: 'Get your nose over your toes'.
- Seat yourself beside the person and lean forwards in an exaggerated way to show him what he has to do.
- Provide a firm pillar of support for the person to push against: the assistant uses her own thigh as a substitute chair arm or to lengthen the chair arm.
- Use the palm-to-palm thumb hold to stop the person from gripping the chair arms.
- Prevent the person from squeezing your hand by using the palm-to-palm thumb hold.

Using two assistants makes some individuals think that you expect the movement to be difficult. They may succeed with one assistant but fail with two.

Note People with a stiff arthritic hip or knee cannot use the normal pattern of rising, they have to use a different one. Someone with a knee that will not bend, slides to the front of the chair in order to get his heel onto the floor before rising. The person whose hip is stiff cannot bend forwards – he has to slide to the front of his chair with his knee bent so that he can place his foot on the floor behind himself.

Throughout give : time

repetition

reassurance

Never pull someone out of his chair.

From Appendix 2 of *Promoting Mobility for People with Dementia:*
A problem-solving approach by Rosemary Oddy.
You may copy these pages.

Chair approach

Aims

- To reduce anxiety.
- To anticipate and manage misjudgements.

Suggested strategies

- Encourage the person to approach the chair across its front using a curved pathway, especially when a walking aid is being used.
- Encourage the person to get his feet beyond the mid-line of chair (the walking aid should be even further ahead) before starting to sit down.
- Allow the person to *keep the chair in sight* and to sit down sideways on it.
- Give little taps to the person's hips to turn him towards the chair (a directional cue).
- Use your own thigh or knee to guide the person's hips safely into the chair.

When someone is helped by two assistants, the one nearer the chair stays behind so that the person's view of the chair is not blocked. This also applies if a lone assistant is on the side that would block the person's view of the chair.

Note The above strategy of sitting down sideways must not be used for someone who is recovering from a recently repaired fractured neck of femur (hip fracture). Following such surgery, sitting down must take place only when the chair is directly behind the person. This means that he cannot see the seat – he is therefore likely to need a great deal of reassurance before he will sit down.

From Appendix 2 of *Promoting Mobility for People with Dementia: A problem-solving approach* by Rosemary Oddy.
You may copy this page.

Walking

General points

- Comfortable footwear.
- Clothes/incontinence pads secure.
- Drainage bags etc hidden.

Suggested strategies

- Walk in unison.
- Aim for a short distance to a seat that the person can see.
- Provide a resting place (chair/stool) half-way.
- Give the walk a purpose (meal, TV, visitor, toilet, exercise).
- Give effective physical support or use a walking aid.
- Make use of the backs of a row of chairs for support/practice.
- Add to the sound of person's feet with your own (sound cue).
- Give the person something to hold in his free hand if he tends to grab the furniture/walls/you/other people.
- Give the person the opportunity to walk longer distances to maintain the 'feel' of the rhythm of walking.
- Reassure the person about the surroundings (hard to soft floor coverings, etc).
- Encourage longer strides by using a 'goose-step' (visual cue).
- If the person's feet shuffle, encourage marching and/or sing a marching tune.
- If the person's feet 'stutter', stop and restart by 'stepping'.
- If the person threatens to sit down on an imaginary chair, tell him firmly 'Stay standing – stand up', and *not* 'Don't sit down'.
- Allow someone who insists on sitting down during a walk to sit on your knee, and then if necessary lower him to the ground.
- Learn the technique of sliding a falling person down your body onto the floor.
- Make walking an enjoyable experience (conversation, attention, etc).
- Make allowances for changes in ability from hour to hour or during the day.

continued

Note If the person leans backwards, discuss this with a physiotherapist. Do not attempt a walk; it could be dangerous.

Never tow a person.

Steps and stairs

General points

- Good lighting is needed.
- Encourage the person to place his whole foot on each tread.
- Make sure that an unsteady or breathless person places one foot onto the tread and then the other (two feet on the same tread) in order to slow him down and allow for better control.
- Use a stout belt round the person's waist to help handling and give him confidence.

Suggested strategies

- Step down the step just ahead of the person, to show the change in level (visual cue).
- Step down the flight of steps or stairs slightly in front of the person, to partially block sight of the space ahead (space-filling strategy).
- Or encourage the person to use both hands on one rail and come down sideways.
- Paint the edge of concrete steps with a wide stripe in a contrasting colour.

Reminder Even if someone does not need to be able to go up and down stairs, he still needs to be able to manage steps.

Transfers

The 'receiving' chair should be positioned close to and at about 90 degrees to the chair the person is sitting on.

Suggested strategies

- Place an extra (third) chair in the space in front of the person (space-filling strategy).
- Demonstrate the side-to-side rocking movement if the person needs to move to the front of the chair (visual cue).
- Tell the person to 'Sit *here*, please' and slap the seat of the chair to make a 'chair noise' (sound cue).
- During the transfer, lightly tap the person's hips in the direction of the receiving chair (touch cue).
- If you are the only assistant, stand in the space between the backs of the two chairs to help the person's hips across more easily.
- If there are two assistants, one of you helps at the person's side and the other from the space between the backs of the two chairs.

Suggested patterns

- Reach across transfer.
- Stand up and then transfer.

Alternative methods

- Use a sliding board and slide the person across.
- Use a weight-bearing hoist if necessary.

Suggested patterns

- Reach across transfer
- Stand up and reach across transfer

From Appendix 2 of *Promoting Mobility for People with Dementia: A problem-solving approach* by Rosemary Oddy.

You may copy this page.

Bed

A FROM LYING TO SITTING ON THE EDGE

This involves major changes of position, so the person needs reassurance and time to adjust to each change.

Suggested strategies

- 'Get up, please' with a rising gesture (visual cue).
- 'Sit on the edge, please' (goal-based request).
- Help the person to roll from lying with knees bent, onto his side; ask him to look at you and to reach for the edge of the bed or your hand.
- Prevent the person from seeing the drop to the floor: block the view and/or place a pillow lengthways along the edge of the bed (space-filling strategy).

B SITTING ON THE EDGE OF THE BED TO LYING DOWN

This is a major change of position.

Suggested strategies

- 'Lie down, please', and slap the pillows to make a 'pillow noise' (sound cue).
- 'Here's the pillow', and help the person to feel it, to encourage lying down along the *length* of the bed (touch cue).
- Ask the person first to lift his legs onto the bed and then to lie down.

C MOVING ACROSS THE BED

Suggested strategies

- 'Move across here, please', with a sliding gesture (directional cue).
- Give guidance with touch cues.
- Use a slide-sheet or doubled plastic bag to help the person's hips across.

Note For A, B and C you may need to accept the person's own safe pattern.

D   MOVING ALONG THE EDGE OF THE BED

Suggested strategies

- 'Move along, please', with a gesture (directional cue).
- Sit beside the person, who uses your thigh as a chair arm; this enables him to raise his hips higher and move sideways more easily.
- Sit beside the person and move up very close against him. Move even closer and ask him to 'Move up/along/across, please' (moving into his personal space).
- Or sit away from the person and pat the bed to encourage him to move towards you, saying 'Come and sit beside me'.

Note   If the person seems to be afraid or unwilling to move, place a chair in the space in front of him, with its back towards him (as used during standing up or transferring).

From Appendix 2 of *Promoting Mobility for People with Dementia: A problem-solving approach* by Rosemary Oddy.

You may copy these pages.

GLOSSARY

carers   the people who are involved in the (unpaid) care of a relative, friend or neighbour.

contractures   the result of muscles or ligaments becoming shortened when they are not regularly stretched by movement

coronary heart disease   a condition in which the arteries to the heart become narrowed

duty of care   having a legal responsibility

ergonomic approach   the job is fitted to the person rather than the person to the job

Lewy body disease   an increasingly recognised type of dementia, which causes frequent variations in behaviour and abilities

load   the person who needs to be assisted to move or the object that has to be lifted

modifications to shoes   professional alterations made to the sole or heel of a shoe to correct a particular problem

osteoporosis   a thinning and weakening of bones, which often leads to fractures; older women are more likely to be affected than older men

Parkinsonism   a condition that often accompanies dementia; it causes stiff muscles (rigidity), unsteadiness, slowness of movement and difficulties in beginning a movement

pattern of movement   the way in which movement is usually carried out; for example, the leaning forwards, raising of hips and straightening up that normally occur when we rise to standing

peripheral vision   what we see to each side of ourselves when we are looking forwards

professional carers   the qualified nurses and care workers and their assistants who are employed to care for people

'sling-backs'   sandals or shoes with a single strap round the back of the heel to hold the sandal or shoe on the wearer's foot

'stuttering' feet   the sudden quick movements of the feet, up and down, experienced by a person with Parkinsonism, that interrupt his normal stride – the heels are raised during the movements and each foot moves only a tiny pace forward.

thrombosis   the formation of a clot of blood that blocks the flow of blood through the affected vein

FURTHER READING

General

Dementia Care: A handbook for residential and day care by Alan Chapman, Alan Jacques and Mary Marshall. Age Concern England, London, 1994

Let's Go Wheelies: Ill-conceived behaviours amongst staff caring for people with dementia by Brian Lodge. BASE (address on p 125), 1992

Person to Person: A guide to those with failing mental powers by Tom Kitwood and Kathleen Bredin. Gale Centre Publications (Whitakers Way, Loughton, Essex IG10 1SQ), 1992

36-Hour Day: A family guide to caring at home for people with Alzheimer's disease and other confusional illnesses by Nancy L Mace and Peter V Rabins. Hodder and Stoughton/Age Concern, London, 1992 [Now out of print but likely to be available from a library]

Working with Dementia by Graham Stokes and Fiona Goudie. Winslow Press (Telford Road, Bicester, Oxon OX6 0TS), 1990

Design, furniture and planning

Carpets: A matter of opinion by Noni Cobban. Dementia Services Development Centre, Stirling (address on p 126), 1994

Chairs: Guidelines for the purchase of lounge, dining and occasional chairs for elderly long-term residents by Janet Wagland and Gretta Peachment. Dementia Services Development Centre, Stirling (address on p 126), 1997

Hard Architecture and Human Scale Designing for Disorientation: A literature review on designing environments for people with dementia by Alan Dunlop. Dementia Services Development Centre, Stirling (address on p 126), 1994

Selecting Easy Chairs: For elderly and disabled people by Caroline Harris and Wendy Mayfield. Institute of Consumer Ergonomics (University of Technology, 75 Swingbridge Road, Loughborough LE11 0JB), 1983

What does 'Barrier Free' Mean for People with Dementia in Designing New Housing by Alison S Smith. Dementia Services Development Centre, Stirling (address on p 126), 1997

Whither Now? Planning Services for People with Dementia by Brian Lodge. BASE (address on p 125), 1991

USEFUL ADDRESSES

Age Concern England

see page 128

Alzheimer's Disease Society

2nd Floor
Gordon House
10 Greencoat Place
London SW1 1PH
Tel: 0171-306 0606

Holds details of local groups; these provide education, support and social events for members (carers of people with dementia, professional workers and interested supporters).

Association of Professional Music Therapists

38 Pierce Lane
Fulbourne
Cambridgeshire CB1 5DL
(please send s.a.e. with any enquiry)

As the professional body for all qualified music therapists in the UK, the Association deals with professional matters and is able to put you in touch with a music therapist if there is one in your area.

BASE (British Association for Services to the Elderly)

119 Hassell Street
Newcastle
Staffordshire ST5 1AX
Tel: 01782 661033

Provides opportunities for professional workers and private individuals who care for older people to meet in an informal atmosphere for an exchange of ideas and experience.

British Society for Music Therapy

25 Rosslin Avenue
East Barnet
Hertfordshire EN4 8DH
(please send s.a.e. with any enquiry)

Supplies general information about music therapy: what it is, how it is applied and what it can achieve.

Carers National Association

20–25 Glasshouse Road
London EC1A 4JS
Tel: 0171-490 8818

Spearheads the campaign for fairer deals for carers and provides them with information on available services.

Chartered Society of Physiotherapy

14 Bedford Row
London WC1R 4ED
Tel: 0171-306 6666

Passes requests for information and queries relating to physiotherapy for people with dementia to the relevant specific interest group.

College of Occupational Therapists

6–8 Marshalsea Road
London SE1 1HL
Tel: 0171-357 6480

Forwards requests for information and queries about occupational therapy for people with dementia to the relevant interest group.

Dementia Services Development Centre

University of Stirling
Stirling FK9 4LA
Tel: 01786 467740

Offers publications for sale: papers, reports and training videos on many aspects of dementia.

Disabled Living Foundation

380–384 Harrow Road
London W9 2HU
Tel: 0171-289 6111

Provides comprehensive information about the range and availability of goods and equipment for 'disabled' people. Able to direct enquirers to their nearest Disabled Living Centre.

King's Fund Centre

11–13 Cavendish Square
London W1N 0AN
Tel: 0171-307 2400

Seeks to promote good practice in health care through research. Offers a forum for informed debate and provides an information service.

Royal College of Nursing (RCN)

20 Cavendish Square
London W1M 0AB
Tel: 0171-409 3333

Booklets on manual handling assessments, codes of practice and handling patients are available from the publications department.

ABOUT AGE CONCERN

Promoting Mobility for People with Dementia: A problem-solving approach is one of a wide range of publications produced by Age Concern England, the National Council on Ageing. Age Concern cares about all older people and believes later life should be fulfilling and enjoyable. For too many this is impossible. As the leading charitable movement in the UK concerned with ageing and older people, Age Concern finds effective ways to change that situation.

Where possible, we enable older people to solve problems themselves, providing as much or as little support as they need. Our network of 1,400 local groups, supported by 250,000 volunteers, provides community-based services such as lunch clubs, day centres and home visiting.

Nationally, we take a leading role in campaigning, parliamentary work, policy analysis, research, specialist information and advice provision, and publishing. Innovative programmes promote healthier lifestyles and provide older people with opportunites to give the experience of a lifetime back to their communities.

Age Concern England is dependent on donations, covenants and legacies.

Age Concern England	**Age Concern Scotland**
1268 London Road	113 Rose Street
London SW16 4ER	Edinburgh EH2 3DT
Tel: 0181-679 8000	Tel: 0131-220 3345

Age Concern Cymru	**Age Concern Northern Ireland**
4th Floor	3 Lower Crescent
1 Cathedral Road	Belfast BT7 1NR
Cardiff CF1 9SD	Tel: 01232 245729
Tel: 01222 371566	

PUBLICATIONS FROM AGE CONCERN BOOKS

Professional, policy & research

Taking Good Care: A handbook for care assistants
Jenyth Worsley

Written for professional carers of older people, *Taking Good Care* discusses the principles and practice of good care. The book's practical approach covers vital communication skills, the role of the care assistant, the medical and social problems of later life and positive activities to keep people feeling fit and part of life.

£7.50   0–86242–072–5

Carefully: A handbook for home care assistants
Lesley Bell

This highly acclaimed and practical guide provides advice on the responsibilities of home care assistants in promoting independence and enabling people to live in their own homes for as long as possible.

£11.99   0–86242–129–2

Dementia Care: A handbook for residential and day care
Alan Chapman, Alan Jacques and Mary Marshall

A comprehensive, practical guide to the delivery of care to people with dementia, this book has been designed for use by those working in both residential and day care settings. It stresses the importance of maintaining respect for people with dementia and upholding their rights as individuals. Topics addressed include:

- understanding the condition
- diagnosis and assessment
- daily care
- coping with unusual behaviour
- legal issues

This handbook provides sound advice on good practice and offers reassurance and support to staff who are often tested to their limits.

£11.99   0–86242–128–4

Reminiscence and Recall: A guide to good practice
Faith Gibson

Designed for use in residential, day and domiciliary care settings, this comprehensive book gives advice on planning and running successful reminiscence work. In addition to detailed background information, the author also provides suggestions for themed topics and advice on intergenerational and life history work. Topics covered include:

- why reminiscence work can be valuable
- how to sustain good practice
- using visual, audio and tactile aids

£11.99   0–86242–142–X

If you would like to order any of these books, please write to the address below, enclosing a cheque or money order for the appropriate amount made payable to Age Concern England. Credit card orders may be made on 0181-679 8000.

Mail Order Unit

Age Concern England
1268 London Road
London SW16 4ER

Information Line

Age Concern produces over 40 comprehensive factsheets designed to answer many of the questions older people – or those advising them – may have, on topics such as:

- finding and paying for residential and nursing home care
- money benefits
- finding help at home
- legal affairs
- making a Will
- help with heating
- raising income from your home
- transfer of assets

Age Concern offers a factsheet subscription service that presents all the factsheets in a folder, together with regular updates throughout the year. The first year's subscription currently costs £50; an annual renewal thereafter is £25.

To order your FREE factsheet list, phone 0800 00 99 66 (a free call) or write to:

Age Concern
FREEPOST (SWB 30375)
Ashburton
Devon TQ13 7ZZ

INDEX